Cigarettes

The First
Comprehensive
Guide to
the Health
Consequences
of Smoking

Cigarettes

What the Warning Label Doesn't Tell You

AMERICAN COUNCIL ON SCIENCE AND HEALTH
FOREWORD BY ELIZABETH M. WHELAN, ACSH PRESIDENT

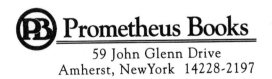
Prometheus Books
59 John Glenn Drive
Amherst, New York 14228-2197

Published 1997 by Prometheus Books

01 00 99 98 97   5 4 3 2 1

Library of Congress Cataloging-in-Publication Data

Cigarettes : what the warning label doesn't tell you : the first comprehensive guide to the health consequences of smoking / from the American Council on Science and Health ; foreward by Elizabeth M. Whelan.
  p.   cm.
Originally published: New York : American Council on Science and Health, 1996.
Previous ed. catalogued under Napier.
Includes bibliographical references and index.
ISBN 1–57392–158–0 (pbk. : alk. paper)
  1. Tobacco—Toxicology. 2. Cigarette habit—Health aspects. 3. Smoking—Health aspects. I. Whelan, Elizabeth M. II. American Council on Science and Health.
RA1242.T6C54   1997
616.86'5—dc21   97–22232
                                                                      CIP

Printed in Canada on acid-free paper

ACKNOWLEDGMENTS

ACSH gratefully acknowledges the comments and contributions of the following individuals who reviewed this report.

STEPHEN BARRETT, M.D., Allentown, Pennsylvania

JOSEPH FRANCIS BORZELLECA, PH.D., Medical College of Virginia

WILLIAM G. CAHAN, M.D., Memorial Sloan-Kettering Cancer Center

ANDREA GOLAINE CASE, M.S.,
American Council on Science and Health

JOEL DUNNINGTON, M.D., M. D. Anderson Cancer Center

JOSEPH ELIA, M.D., Reno, Nevada

RAYMOND GAMBINO, M.D., Corning Clinical Laboratories

K. H. GINZEL, M.D., University of Arkansas for Medical Sciences

CLARK W. HEATH, JR., M.D., American Cancer Society

THOMAS HOUSTON, M.D., American Medical Association

WILLIAM M. LONDON, ED.D., M.P.H.,
American Council on Science and Health

W. K. C. MORGAN, M.D., London Health Sciences Centre, Ontario

ALBERT G. NICKEL, Lyons Lavey Nickel Swift, Inc.

R. T. RAVENHOLT, M.D., M.P.H., Population Health Imperatives

DONALD SHOPLAND, National Cancer Institute (NCI)
Smoking and Tobacco Control Program

JOHN SLADE, M.D., Robert Wood Johnson Medical School

FREDRICK J. STARE, M.D., P.H.D., Harvard School of Public Health

MICHAEL THUN, M.D., American Cancer Society

ROBERT P. UPCHURCH, PH.D., University of Arizona

ELIZABETH M. WHELAN, SC.D., M.P.H.,
American Council on Science and Health

JOEL ELLIOT WHITE, M.D., Walnut Creek, California

ROBERT J. WHITE, M.D., PH.D., Case Western Reserve University
School of Medicine, MetroHealth Medical Center

ACSH gratefully acknowledges the comments and contributions of the following individuals who reviewed specific chapters related to their medical specialty fields.

WILMA BERGFELD, M.D., The Cleveland Clinic Foundation; Past
President, American Academy of Dermatologists (Smoking and the Skin)

RUSSELL CECIL, M.D., Orthopedic Surgeon, Amsterdam, New York
(Smoking and Orthopedic Problems)

EMIL W. CHYNN, M.D., Emory University Department of
Ophthalmology, Atlanta, Georgia (Smoking and the Eyes)

STEPHEN K. EPSTEIN, M.D., M.P.P., Associate in Medicine, Harvard
Medical School; Division of Emergency Medicine, Beth Israel Hospital,
Boston, Massachusetts (Smoking and Emergency Medicine)

FREDERICK L. FERRIS, M.D., National Eye Institute (Smoking and the Eyes)

ACKNOWLEDGMENTS

CARMEN FONSECA, M.D., Department of Vascular Medicine, The Cleveland Clinic Foundation (Smoking and Peripheral Vascular Disease)

CARYL GUTH, M.D, Anesthesiologist, Mills-Peninsula Hospital, San Mateo, California (Smoking and Surgical Risk)

ROBERT G. LAHITA, M.D., Ph.D., Associate Professor, Columbia University; Chief of Rheumatology, St. Luke's-Roosevelt Medical Center, New York, New York (Smoking and Rheumatologic Conditions)

ARNOLD LEVINSON, M.D., University of Pennsylvania, Philadelphia, Pennsylvania (Smoking and the Immune System)

JANET MACHLEDT, M.D., M.S., M.P.H., Texas Oncology, P.A., Houston, Texas (Oncology: Smoking and Cancer Risk)

HELEN GARDNER MARTIN, M.D., Northwestern University School of Medicine (Smoking and Lung Disease)

STEPHEN J. MOSS, D.D.S., M.S., David B. Kriser Dental Center, New York, New York (Smoking and Oral Health)

HARRIS M. NAGLER, M.D., Chairman, Department of Urology, Beth Israel Medical Center, New York, New York; Professor of Urology, The Albert Einstein College of Medicine, Bronx, New York (Smoking and Urology: Male Fertility and Sexuality Dysfunctions)

DAVID R. NIELSEN, M.D., Southwest Otologic Institute, Ltd., Phoenix, Arizona (Otolaryngology: Abnormalities of the Ears, Nose and Throat Associated with Smoking)

JOHN PATRICK O'GRADY, M.D., Director of Obstetrical Services, Chief of Maternal Fetal Medicine, Professor of Obstetrics and Gynecology, Baystate Medical Center, Springfield, Massachusetts; Professor of Obstetrics and Gynecology, Tufts University School of Medicine, Boston, Massachusetts (Smoking and Complications in Obstetrics and Gynecology)

---

*ACSH would also like to thank The Commonwealth Fund, a New York
City–based national foundation undertaking independent research on health
and social issues, for their generous support of this project.*

TABLE OF CONTENTS

Cigarettes: The Undisclosed Medical Risks

As popular (and deadly) as they are today, cigarettes weren't even viable commercial products in the United States until about 1915. Up to that time, tobacco had commonly been smoked in pipes or cigars or had been used in its smokeless forms. Tobacco in those forms presented real health hazards, but it became uniquely dangerous to health as cigarettes emerged.

The cigarette—along with its critical accompaniment, the portable, easy-to-light match, also a product of this century—offered two notable "advantages" over other tobacco products. First, the cigarette allowed tobacco and its associated chemicals and fibers to be inhaled easily. Second, it provided the opportunity for a "quick smoke" anytime and anywhere, as opposed, for example, to the ritual after-dinner smoking of a cigar or a pipe, lit from a candle or a taper held to the fire.

Disturbing medical reports—particularly a startling increase in lung cancer, until then a relatively rare disease—began to abound in the 1930s. The reports increased in the 1940s. By the early 1950s the "real" proof of cigarettes' contribution to lung cancer and heart disease risk was there. The public and private "controversy" about whether or not cigarettes were a hazard to health ended officially in 1964 with the release of the first United States Surgeon General's report.[1]

After the appearance of the Surgeon General's report, national public opinion polls confirmed that the overwhelming majority of Americans said that they knew cigarette smoking was "dangerous." Following the placement of a federally mandated health "warning" label on cigarette packs in 1966 and on cigarette advertisements in 1969, the evolving popular wisdom became, "Everyone knows the health hazards of smoking; and smokers know the risks they're assuming—see, it's right here on the label."

This popular wisdom has now become the mantra of those who oppose litigation against cigarette companies. It serves as a guiding principle for the people who reject calls for more responsible action on the part of the cigarette industry and for more government oversight of the industry's business practices.

In this book the American Council on Science and Health (ACSH) directly challenges this widely held bit of popular wisdom. ACSH believes that in 1996 Americans—smokers and nonsmokers alike—have only the most cursory understanding of the extent and magnitude of the health risks associated with cigarette smoking as compared with other alleged health risks in the environment.

Normally, when products are marketed in the United States, their manufacturers are legally responsible for keeping abreast of the latest scientific and medical data concerning the safety of those products. Tort law requires manufacturers to keep consumers fully informed about real or potential health risks associated with their products. A manufacturer who detects a defect that might harm consumers—a defect in, say, an automobile, a lawnmower or a baby carriage—has an economic incentive to notify customers—even to recall a product—if the manufacturer suspects a hazard exists or identifies a new hazard. The incentive to warn consumers is provided by the ever-present threat of future litigation against the manufacturer by a consumer who suffers harm from the product. This threat of litigation is a strong motivator to keep manufacturers up to date and forthcoming on the medical risks, if any, of their products.

Cigarette manufacturers enjoy a unique legal status, however, and so have no such incentive to report risks. When the United States Congress mandated the so-called "Surgeon General's Warning Label" on cigarette packs and advertisements, it simultaneously excused the tobacco industry from any obligation to warn consumers in detail about the dangers of those products. Congress in effect "preempted" the responsibility of the cigarette manufacturers to provide a detailed warning.

Smokers and would-be smokers in the years from 1964 to the present might have known in the rhetorical sense that smoking was "dangerous"; but they did not—and still do not—have some essential pieces of information that would allow them to make a truly informed decision whether or not to smoke. *This information should have been provided by the industry but never was.* Although many people take up smoking because they find an allure in the self-destruction it offers, this behavior does not excuse the cigarette industry from its ethical responsibility to give consumers adequate information about the full range and magnitude of smoking's risks.

To be truly informed, a consumer needs the answers to a number of basic questions:

1. **"What is the safe level of cigarette smoking?" or, to put it another way, "What is the upper limit of the number of cigarettes I can smoke before I begin to incur health risks?"**

What the scientific literature says:
It is difficult at this point to identify a "no-hazard" level of smoking. As will be clear from the pages that follow, transient physiological effects of smoking, particularly on the cardiovascular system, are identifiable after one cigarette. While it is possible that smoking just a few cigarettes a day might not present a significant health risk to most people, there are relatively few smokers who limit their smoking that much. The vast majority of current smokers smoke more than 15 cigarettes a day[2]—clearly a level that dramatically increases the risk of many diseases.

What the cigarette industry and the Congressionally mandated warning label disclose to consumers:
Neither the industry nor the warning label has ever warned consumers that smoking is exceptionally addictive or has pointed out the minimum amount of smoking that poses health hazards. In comparison, the manufacturers of alcoholic beverages and the government, through various publications on the health effects of alcohol, have for decades called for "moderation" in the consumption of alcohol. Further, both industry and government have defined (with some variation) what moderation is: It is in the range of from one to three ounces of 80-proof alcohol or its equivalent in wine or beer.

2. **"What specifically are the potential health hazards associated with cigarette smoking?"**

What the scientific literature says:
As this book details, cigarette smoking is known to adversely affect nearly every system and function of the human body. Cigarette smoking causes malignancies and adverse effects on organs that have no direct contact

with the smoke itself. It increases the risk of cancers of the pancreas, the bladder, the colon and the cervix. It is also a causative factor in male impotence, infertility, blindness, hearing loss and bone loss.

What the industry and the label disclose:
As recently as 1994, when the chief executive officers of the major cigarette manufacturers testified before Congress, the industry has denied knowledge of any health risks associated with cigarette smoking.

The various rotating, mandated warning labels note an increased risk of cancer, heart disease and various lung diseases as well as "complications" in pregnancy. The details of the risks—including the sites at which cancer risk is increased and the other common health consequences of smoking that go beyond cancer, heart disease and lung disease—have never been presented by the industry. Neither have they been disclosed on the mandated labels.

By way of contrast, take a look at any of the many multipage advertisements for prescription drugs that appear almost weekly in such consumer magazines as *TV Guide* and *Parade*. The first page of such an ad is usually a glossy encomium for the product, laid out in a style familiar to readers of over-the-counter drug and cosmetic ads. But turn the page and you find a detailed list in tiny print of contraindications, precautions and specifics of "what could go wrong," including unlikely hazards. It's a far cry from the discreetly unobtrusive Surgeon General's warnings, which have come to be regarded as merely another bit of visual "snow." Readers have learned to ignore these minimally intrusive little boxes just as they've learned to ignore the UPC-code boxes snuggled into the corners of their favorite magazines' covers.

3. "What is the relative magnitude of the various risks associated with smoking cigarettes?"

We live in an age of warning labels. The artificial sweetener saccharin carries a label warning that it causes cancer in laboratory animals. Cups of fast-food coffee warn us that the liquid is hot and could cause a burn. The media tell us about the alleged "carcinogen of the week"— Alar on apples, nitrite in bacon. Everything seems to cause cancer or otherwise threaten our health. Where do cigarettes fit into the scheme of dangerous things?

What the scientific literature says:
Cigarette smoking is by far the leading cause of preventable death in the United States. It is responsible for approximately 500,000 deaths each year.[3] About one death in four—one death in two designated as "premature"—is attributable to smoking. A recent study concluded that even among people admitted for inpatient treatment of alcoholism and other non-nicotine drug dependencies, tobacco-related causes of death are significantly more frequent than alcohol-related causes.[4]

The concept of "risk" is a tricky one for consumers. The risk of drinking apple juice prepared from Alar-exposed apples is purely hypothetical. We have no studies of humans that suggest such a risk exists. But we do have an overwhelming number of studies that indicate that pack-a-day smokers, when compared with people who have never smoked, have 10 times the risk of lung cancer and twice the risk of heart disease. (Although smoking increases the risk of death from lung cancer more dramatically than it increases the risk of death from coronary heart disease, smokers in the United States die from coronary heart disease slightly more often than they do from lung cancer.[5] A doubling of the risk of death from coronary heart disease, a common cause of death among nonsmokers, yields a slightly higher number than does a tenfold increase in lung cancer, a relatively rare disease among nonsmokers.)

What the industry and the label disclose:
Cigarette companies and the Congressionally mandated label have never defined the extent of the risks assumed by smoking; nor have they contrasted those risks with the everyday risks of life, such as crossing a busy street.

4. "Are the risks of smoking reversible, and if so, at what age?"

What the scientific literature says:
Many, if not most, smokers assume that they will eventually give up the habit. They also assume that when they do, their health-risk profile will return to normal.

While quitting smoking brings substantial health benefits at any age, the literature points to "threshold" amounts of smoking that produce irreversible increases in risk for some diseases. Quitting can prevent the risk from increasing further, but the prior cumulative exposure can have permanent consequences. For example, two 1994 reports in the *Journal of the National Cancer Institute* indicate that for both men and women, smoking a pack a day for 10 to 14 years appears to double irreversibly the risk of developing colon cancer decades later.[6,7]

What the industry and the label disclose:
Neither has ever provided any information to consumers about the timing and nature of the irreversible health risks of cigarette smoking.

5. "Considering the adverse health effects of smoking, is there a way I might monitor my health to detect any possible damage earlier rather than later"?

What the scientific literature says:
Screening for early detection of a number of diseases—such as cervical cancer—for which smoking is a risk factor is advisable for smokers and nonsmokers alike. There are, however, also some early-detection checks that may be advisable for smokers that may not be necessary for nonsmokers. For example, in 1989 the U.S. Preventive Services Task Force did not recommend routine screening for peripheral arterial disease (PAD) in asymptomatic persons, but the task force noted that clinicians should be alert to signs of PAD in persons at increased risk—such as smokers. And while the task force did not recommend routine electrocardiography in asymptomatic persons for reducing the risk of coronary artery disease, it noted that screening electrocardiography may be clinically prudent for asymptomatic males over age 40 with two or more cardiac risk factors—of which one might be smoking.[8]

What the industry and the label disclose:
Neither the industry nor the mandated label has ever warned cigarette smokers to monitor their health for early and perhaps reversible signs of cigarette-related illness. In contrast, a number of prescription drugs now on the market, while deemed "safe" and effective for use, carry warnings

of potential undesirable health consequences—such as damage to the liver—and recommendations for surveillance—such as regular liver-function tests—to assess the drugs' impact.

6. "Do cigarettes interact adversely with other products to intensify the negative health risks?"

Recently, manufacturers of over-the-counter pain killers have suggested that consumers who enjoy more than three or four alcoholic drinks a day might want to discuss with their doctors their use of the pain killers. These suggestions are based on concerns about a "synergism" of the pain killers and the alcohol—a combined action with a total effect greater than that of either the pain killers or the alcohol when taken alone. Such an interaction could cause problems that might not occur if only one of the products were used.

What the scientific literature says:
It has been clear for decades that there is an enormous negative synergism between cigarette smoking and the consumption of alcoholic beverages. For example, smokers who regularly consume alcoholic beverages have a truly spectacular increased probability of developing esophageal cancer. If these consumers smoked but didn't drink, or drank but didn't smoke, their risk of cancer at that particular site would be substantially reduced.[9]

What the industry and the label disclose:
Neither the industry nor the mandated warning label has ever disclosed the enormous synergistic effect alcohol consumption has on esophageal cancer among cigarette smokers.

7. "Have there been any new risks of smoking identified since the Surgeon General's report in 1964?"

What the scientific literature says:
There are over 70,000 medical articles detailing the dangers of smoking. As this book notes, new findings since 1964 have implicated cigarette smoking as a causal factor in a wide range of ailments. Even during the

1990s new causal information has continued to be identified; researchers at the National Cancer Institute have identified cigarette smoking as a causal factor in colon cancer, for example.

What the industry and the label disclose:
There has never been an attempt on the part of either the industry or the Congress to keep consumers apprised of the growing list of diseases causally associated with cigarette smoking.

8. **"Is there any other information I should have that will allow me to be an informed consumer when I decide whether or not to start or continue smoking?"**

What the scientific literature says:
The United States Surgeon General has determined that cigarette smoking is addictive and that the pharmacological and behavioral processes that determine tobacco addiction are similar to those that determine addiction to other drugs, such as heroin and cocaine. Nicotine is the psychoactive drug in tobacco that reinforces its continued use. According to a study published in the *Journal of the American Medical Association*, cocaine addicts in treatment tended to find cigarettes harder to give up than cocaine.[10]

What the industry and the label disclose:
The industry has long denied that either cigarette smoking or nicotine is addictive and has effectively opposed any attempt to include that information on the mandated label.

In recent years there has been an increase in the volume of the public debate and an increase in the controversy over what can be done, within a free society, to reduce the burden of cigarette-related disease and death. The American Council on Science and Health and other advocacy groups have long taken an aggressive and unwavering position on the dangers of smoking. Critics have dismissed antismoking groups as "health Nazis" and "health nannies"—repressive killjoys who want to control how people live and deny them their basic "freedom" to smoke.

ACSH enthusiastically promotes an individual's freedom to make lifestyle choices. But freedom is only achievable when the choice is truly informed; and ACSH believes that as we approach the 21st century, the decision to start smoking is rarely a truly informed one. Three thousand children under the age of 18 take up smoking every day.[11] Considering the powerful pharmacological and behavioral factors influencing smoking addiction, the claim that smokers are celebrants of individual freedom should be treated with skepticism.

If indeed "the truth will make us free," perhaps the following 20 chapters of full disclosure of the medical effects of smoking will serve as the first milestones along the road toward true freedom of choice. ACSH scientists have prepared this relatively brief volume to increase public knowledge of the health risks of smoking. But having begun the process, we would like to return the responsibility to those to whom it properly belongs: the manufacturers of cigarettes.

ELIZABETH M. WHELAN
President
American Council on Science and Health
New York, New York
August 1996

References

1   Department of Health, Education, and Welfare. *Smoking and Health. Report of the Advisory Committee to the Surgeon General of the Public Health Service.* Washington, DC: US Department of Health, Education, and Welfare; 1964. Public Health Service publication 1103.

2   Pierce JP, Hatziandreu E, Flyer P, et al. *Tobacco use in 1996—Methods and Basic Tabulations from Adult Use of Tobacco Survey.* Rockville, MD:Office on Smoking and Health; 1989. US Department of Health and Human Services publication OM 90-2004. Cited in: Novotny TE. Tobacco use. In: Brownson RC, Remington PL, Davis JR, eds. *Chronic Disease Epidemiology and Control.* Washington, DC: American Public Health Association; 1993.

3   Peto R, Lopez AD, Boreham J, Thun M, Heath, Jr., C. *Mortality from Smoking in Developed Countries 1950–2000: Indirect Estimates from National Vital Statistics.* Oxford: Oxford University Press; 1994:211.

4   Hurt RD, Offord KP, Croghan IT, et al. Mortality following inpatient addictions treatment: role of tobacco use in a community-based cohort. *JAMA* 1996; 275:1097–1103.

5   Savitz DA, Harris RP, Brownson RC. Methods in chronic disease epidemiology. In Brownson RC, Remington PL, Davis JR, eds. *Chronic Disease Epidemiology and Control.* Washington, DC: American Public Health Association; 1993.

6   Giovannucci E, Rimm ER, Stampfer MJ, et al. A prospective study of cigarette smoking and risk of colorectal adenoma and colorectal cancer in US men. *J Natl Cancer Inst* 1994; 86:183–191.

7   Giovannucci E, Colditz GA, Stampfer MJ et al. A prospective study of cigarette smoking and risk of colorectal adenoma and colorectal cancer in US women. *J Natl Cancer Inst* 1994; 86:192–199.

8   U.S. Preventive Services Task Force. *Guide to Clinical Preventive Services: A Guide of the Effectiveness of 169 Interventions.* Baltimore, MD: Williams & Wilkins; 1989.

9   Newcomb PA, Carbone PP. The health consequences of smoking: cancer. *Med Clin North Am* 1992; 76:305–331.

10 Kozlowski LT, Wilkinson DA, Skinner W, Kent C, Franklin T, Pope M. Comparing tobacco cigarette dependence with other drug dependencies: greater or equal 'difficulty quitting' and 'urges to use,' but less pleasure from cigarettes. *JAMA* 1989; 261:898–901.

11 Committee on Preventing Nicotine Addiction in Children and Youths, Division of Biobehavioral Sciences and Mental Disorders, Institute of Medicine; Lynch BS, Bonnie RJ, eds. *Growing Up Tobacco Free: Preventing Nicotine Addiction in Children and Youths.* Washington, DC: National Academy Press; 1994.

PREFACE

Cigarette smoking is not just our leading cause of premature death. As best-selling author Fletcher Knebel is said to have quipped, "Smoking is one of the leading causes of statistics." This book confirms how right he was. *Cigarettes: What the Warning Label Doesn't Tell You* discusses numerous studies showing that cigarette smoking is statistically associated with numerous health problems. A statistical association is not, however, the same as a cause-and-effect relationship. Thus, before concluding that smoking or any other activity causes a particular disease, public health researchers consider all pertinent evidence in the context of accepted standards, as discussed in the Introduction that follows.

Using this approach, researchers have found cigarette smoking guilty beyond a reasonable doubt of causing myriad health problems—ranging from the cosmetic (e.g., skin wrinkling) to the deadly (e.g., lung cancer), and from the familiar (e.g., coronary heart disease) to the esoteric (e.g., *thromboangiitis obliterans*). This approach may not offer absolute proof; but there is no need for absolute proof, as three epidemiologists recently noted:

> . . . the tobacco companies argue that the association between smoking and disease is uncertain. In a technical sense, we will always have some degree of uncertainty, especially with no definitive data from large numbers of subjects randomly assigned to be smokers and nonsmokers. We have no doubt, however, that the evidence indicates a need to intervene, because smoking has no clear health benefits and scientists have exhausted all reasonable noncausal explanations for the strong associations observed between smoking and a number of diseases.[1]

As *Cigarettes* makes clear, for some diseases that are statistically associated with cigarette smoking, the evidence is not sufficient to conclude that smoking is a causal factor. To give just one example, some reports suggest that cigarette smoking may worsen retinopathy, the common eye complication of diabetes. Chapter 15 notes the limitations of the evidence implicating smoking in this instance. Accelerated development of diabetic retinopathy is probably better characterized as a suspected, rather than an established, health effect of cigarette smoking.

Cigarettes also discusses evidence suggesting that smoking may have protective effects against the development of some conditions such as Parkinson's disease and Alzheimer's disease. But, as noted in Chapter 13, there are reasonable alternative explanations that might account for these reported epidemiologic associations; and any possible beneficial effects of smoking are dwarfed by the habit's detrimental impacts.

Table 1 (pages xix–xxii) lists both established and suspected health effects of cigarette smoking that are discussed in each chapter of the book. I offer this table as a starting point for cigarette companies which, in fairness to their customers, should be interested in developing a warning label that fully discloses the specifics of how cigarette smoking is hazardous to your health.

WILLIAM M. LONDON
Director of Public Health
American Council on Science and Health
New York, August 1996

TABLE I: SELECTED ESTABLISHED AND SUSPECTED HEALTH EFFECTS OF CIGARETTE SMOKING DISCUSSED IN EACH CHAPTER

CHAPTER	ESTABLISHED AND SUSPECTED EFFECTS
1 **Smoking and Lung Disease**	lung cancer; chronic obstructive lung disease; increased severity of asthma; increased risk of developing various respiratory infections
2 **Oncology: Smoking and Cancer Risk**	esophageal, laryngeal, oral, bladder, kidney, stomach, pancreatic, vulvular, cervical and colorectal cancers
3 **Smoking and Heart Disease**	coronary heart disease; *angina pectoris;* heart attack; repeat heart attack; arrhythmia; aortic aneurysm; cardiomyopathy
4 **Smoking and Peripheral Vascular Disease**	peripheral vascular disease; *thromboangiitis obliterans*
5 **Smoking and the Skin**	wrinkling; fingernail discoloration; psoriasis; palmoplantar pustulosis

Reference

1   Savitz DA, Harris RP, Brownson RC Methods in chronic disease epidemiology. In Brownson RC, Remington PL, Davis JR *Chronic Disease Epidemiology and Control* Washington: American Public Health Association, 1993, p. 31.

The Leading Cause of Preventable Death

Cigarette smoke is the leading cause of preventable death. It kills approximately 500,000 Americans each year, and many more suffer from smoking-related illnesses caused by both direct smoking and exposure to secondhand smoke.

Most people know that smoking is the single most important cause of lung cancer. Many are aware that smoking contributes to other respiratory conditions, but few are aware of the variety and wide range of smoking-associated health problems.

The government-mandated health warnings on cigarette packs and in advertisements offer meager accounts of the health consequences of smoking. The grim reality is that no system of a smoker's body is spared smoking's deleterious effects. Smoking is a major cause of heart disease, stroke, impotence, hearing loss, impaired vision, loss of bone density and other maladies. Taken together, the full spectrum of diseases causally linked with smoking can be described collectively as "tobaccosis."

While national polls indicate that nearly 90 percent of Americans "know" that smoking is hazardous, they know it only in a superficial sense. We are flooded by health warnings today: warnings against artificial sweeteners ("saccharin causes cancer in laboratory animals"), coffee ("restaurant coffee is hot; you can burn yourself if you spill it") and even appliances (refrigerators carry a label noting that the cooling apparatus contains chemicals that can harm health). In today's complex world it is not difficult to misjudge the relative importance of various risks.

In this book, "the devil is in the details." In these pages we provide detailed information on the health effects of smoking, with each chapter addressing effects viewed by a different medical specialty field. The information underscores the stark fact that cigarettes are unique in their malignant effects: They are the only legally available product that is harmful *when used as intended.* The pervasiveness of their destructive effects on health and life thus exceeds that of any other widely used, legally available product in the world today.

Within seconds after tobacco smoke is inhaled, some 4,000 toxic byproducts are absorbed into the bloodstream and transported to every cell of the smoker's body. Nicotine and other ingredients in tobacco can be measured in such seemingly remote body tissues as seminal fluid, cervical secretions, the eyes and the hair.

Some of the smoking-related conditions described in this book are relatively rare, even in smokers. And everyone knows at least one smoker "who has smoked for 40 years and is healthy as a horse." But consider an analogy: Two soldiers must each traverse a field. Soldier A has to cross a field laden with land mines; soldier B, a field relatively free of such deadly traps. While each soldier may indeed cross his field safely, the odds definitely favor soldier B. Soldier A may succeed in avoiding many—maybe even most—of the land mines; but he is highly unlikely to avoid all of them.

Similarly, a smoker may live a long life, avoiding one tobacco-associated disease or cancer after another. But the chances of suffering health problems attributable to smoking are great, and those chances increase both with the length of time the person smokes and with the amount smoked. Cigarette smoking is not only the leading cause of preventable death in the United States today; it is also the leading cause of preventable early ill health and disability.

The American Council on Science and Health (ACSH) has prepared this book as a primer to inform participants in the public policy debate about cigarettes. Public health professionals, health care providers and antismoking activists will find the book to be a unique reference source regarding the hazards of cigarette smoking.

In view of the grave importance of the subject matter in this book, we at ACSH wanted to present readers with a report of the highest caliber. To that end, each chapter of this book has been researched carefully and then reviewed and signed by an expert in the corresponding field of medicine. ACSH is grateful for the assistance of these reviewers and also for the suggestions offered by additional experts who reviewed this report for accuracy, comprehensiveness and readability.

Methods Used to Study Risk of Disease in People
Researchers cannot conduct controlled experiments to test whether or not smoking causes disease, as it is unethical to force people to smoke and then wait to see if they get sick. Rather, scientists rely on epidemiologic, or population-based, studies to suggest and then establish an association. To do this, researchers compare one group of people who have a certain

risk factor—in this case, smoking—with a similar group of people who don't have the risk factor—in this case, nonsmokers. This latter group is called the control group. The subjects in the control group are chosen to be as similar as possible to the smokers in many characteristics, such as age, sex and health status.

Researchers also take into account other factors that may contribute to the development of the disease being studied. For example, when testing whether or not smoking causes oral cancer, researchers must "control" for the use of alcohol, which, when consumed in excess, also raises cancer risk.

Researchers have several yardsticks against which they judge whether the available scientific evidence is strong enough to infer that a risk factor causes a certain disease and is not merely statistically associated with it. Those yardsticks include:[1]

- *Consistency:* Do many different studies and types of studies show the same or consistent results?

- *Strength of the association:* Is the risk associated with the exposure high enough to cause a significant number of new cancer cases (in other words, is the relative risk greater than one)?

- *Biologic gradient:* Is there a dose response? Does the risk depend on the intensity of the exposure (in other words, does the risk increase as the degree of exposure increases)?

- *Temporality:* Did the exposure occur prior to disease onset? In the case of cigarette smoking, there appears to be a 10- to 20-year lag time before cancers begin to develop.

- *Plausibility:* Does the proposed mechanism make sense from a scientific point of view (in other words, does the induction of cancer make sense from what we know about the biologic actions of cigarette smoke)?

KRISTINE NAPIER
August, 1996

Reference

1 Hill AB. The environment and disease: association or causation. *Proc Royal Soc Med.* 1965; 58:295–300.

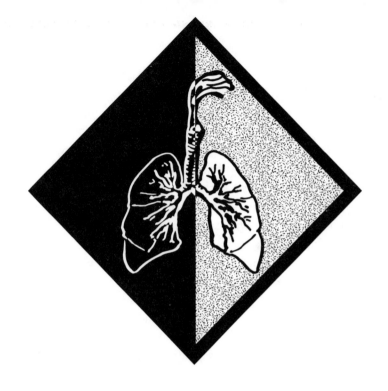

Chapter 1

SMOKING

AND LUNG DISEASE

reviewed by
Helen Gardner Martin, M.D.
Associate Professor of Medicine
Northwestern University
School of Medicine
Chicago, Illinois

It's been over 30 years since the U.S. Surgeon General announced that smoking causes lung disease. Today we know that cigarette smoking is the leading cause not only of lung cancer but also of all pulmonary illness and death in the United States. One researcher has described cigarette smoking as causing "a chronic inflammatory disorder of the lower airways."[1]

While lung cancer is the most well-known smoking-induced lung disease, it is just one of many such ailments from which smokers suffer. Smokers also have greatly increased risks for emphysema and chronic bronchitis, collectively known as chronic obstructive pulmonary disease (COPD). Smoking, in fact, is the most important factor in causing COPD: It is responsible for 90 percent of all cases of emphysema.

Asthmatics who continue to smoke suffer worse forms of the disease. Infectious diseases that affect the lung—including pneumonia, tuberculosis, influenza and the common cold—are generally more severe and more persistent in smokers. Overall, smoking is responsible for over 84,000 annual deaths due to lung diseases other than cancer, including pneumonia, influenza, bronchitis and emphysema.[1,2]

In this chapter we review how smoking affects lung function and then discuss in more detail the smoking-induced lung diseases common among smokers.

How Smoking Affects Lung Function

As a prelude to understanding what happens in smokers' lungs, let's take a look at the respiratory system. When we breathe, air enters the upper airway through the nose and mouth, where the air is filtered, warmed and humidified. The inhaled air then travels through the trachea, or windpipe, to the lungs. Inside each lung there is a main stem, the bronchus, that is analogous to the main stalk in a bunch of grapes. The tiny "stems" running off the "stalk" are called bronchioles. The bronchioles lead, finally, to little air sacs, called alveoli, that look like clusters of grapes. It is in the alveoli that air exchange takes place. Oxygen is exchanged for carbon dioxide in the blood; the blood then carries oxygen to all the body's tissues.

The respiratory system has several built-in safeguards to protect it against disease. The filtering that takes place in the upper airway helps prevent infectious and irritating substances from entering the lung. The trachea and lung tissue produce mucus, which helps trap and carry away contaminants. The mucus-contaminant mix is moved through the lungs by tiny hairs called cilia that beat rapidly back and forth—in some areas, at a rate of up to 1,000 times per minute. When smoke is inhaled through the mouth, smokers automatically bypass the first safeguard, the filtering action of the nose. While smokers often produce more mucus in response to smoking, they are less able than nonsmokers to move the mucus out of their respiratory systems. This happens because cigarette smoking paralyzes and eventually destroys cilia. It also changes the makeup of the mucus-secreting glands and consequently the mucus itself. In addition, mucus glands sometimes become plugged and less able to produce mucus. The end result is that smokers' mucus, contaminated with potentially harmful substances, is more likely to become trapped in the lung tissue.

Additional physical changes in smokers' lung tissue impair the lungs' ability to take in oxygen. Smoking destroys the alveoli, making the lungs less elastic and less able to exchange oxygen. Smokers' lungs also have decreased surface area and fewer capillaries, which means they have decreased blood flow. This robs both lung and body tissues of the nutrients and oxygen they need to be healthy and to function normally.

Smoking also causes a phenomenon called *airway hyperresponsiveness*. In response to the noxious chemicals in tobacco smoke, the airway in effect clamps down. When this happens, the smoker has a greater difficulty getting air in and out of the lungs and so will wheeze and eventually feel short of breath.

These physical changes in the lung result in several other functional changes. To understand those changes, one must understand how to measure lung function. Of the many measurements available, one is *forced expiratory volume in one second* (FEV_1)—the amount of air exhaled during the first second of expiration. Smokers have, among other abnormalities, a greatly reduced FEV_1.[3]

The carbon monoxide in inhaled cigarette smoke binds to hemoglobin, the oxygen-carrying molecule in the blood, to form carboxyhemoglobin. That means there is less hemoglobin available to carry and deliver oxygen to the body's cells. This explains why smokers experience shortness of breath on physical exertion; sometimes, even at rest.

Smoking impairs lung growth and lung tissue maturation in children and adolescents. Another type of lung-growth impairment occurs in smokers aged 20 to 40. During this stage of life, the lungs undergo a type of growth called the plateau phase. This phase is shortened in smokers, which shortens the latency period, or the time with which tobacco-induced diseases develop. Thus, smokers who take up smoking at younger ages are more apt to suffer smoking-related disease after shorter periods of time than are smokers who begin smoking later in life.[4]

Lung Cancer

Smoking accounts for the overwhelming majority of lung cancer cases—some 87 percent of the estimated 177,000 new cases expected in 1996.[5] On average, smokers multiply their risk of contracting lung cancer by five to 10 times.[6] Further, because only about 13 percent of lung cancer patients survive more than five years, smoking is also responsible for the bulk of lung cancer deaths: For 1996 an estimated 90 percent, or 85,000 lung cancer deaths in men, and an estimated 79 percent, or 51,000 lung cancer deaths in women, will be attributable to smoking.[5]

Male smokers are about 22 times more likely than those who have never smoked to die of lung cancer; female smokers have a risk that is about 12 times greater.[5] And while many women believe breast cancer to be the most common cause of cancer death among women, in 1988 lung cancer surpassed breast cancer as the leading cause of cancer death in women.[5]

Rates of lung cancer have increased dramatically over the past 60 years, and the rates show a close association with increases in the number of cigarettes smoked. In fact, lung cancer rates have increased much more than have the rates of any other major type of cancer; and lung cancer is now the most common fatal malignancy in the United States (skin cancer is more common, but it is fatal much less often).[5]

How much must someone smoke to increase his or her risk of lung cancer? At present, it appears that any amount of smoking increases risk. In other words, there is no established threshold or minimum amount necessary to cause cancer.[1] But one thing is clear: Cancer risk does increase with increasing pack-years of smoking. (The pack-year is a measure of overall cigarette consumption—"twenty pack-years" is the equivalent of smoking two packs a day for 10 years or one pack a day for 20 years.) Research has also demonstrated that the younger someone begins smoking, the more likely that person is to get lung cancer.

Chronic Obstructive Pulmonary Disease: Emphysema and Chronic Bronchitis

Chronic obstructive pulmonary disease (COPD) is a generic term used by clinicians to refer to lung damage associated with air-flow obstruction. The two main types of COPD are emphysema and chronic bronchitis. Cigarette smoking is the single most important cause of both chronic bronchitis and emphysema; it accounts for almost all cases of both.[7] The association of COPD with smoking is almost as strong as the lung cancer–smoking association.[1]

Cigarette smoking also makes other risk factors for these chronic conditions more potent. In particular, smokers are more adversely affected by air pollution, infections and occupational exposures such as noxious fumes and asbestos than are nonsmokers.

COPD is fatal in smokers more often than it is in nonsmokers; in fact, smokers are 10 times more likely to die of COPD than are nonsmokers. Overall, cigarette smoking accounts for 82 percent of the annual 80,000 COPD deaths.[7]

Emphysema affects approximately 1.6 million Americans. The disease develops over many years of continuous exposure to a noxious substance—in most cases, cigarette smoke.[7] In people who have emphysema, alveoli in the lung break down. When this happens, the air compartments become abnormally enlarged; eventually the lungs lose their elasticity and become unable to contract normally during expiration. Over time, people who suffer from emphysema grow short of breath and may eventually become totally dependent on supplemental oxygen delivered from a tank. The damage characteristic of emphysema is not reversible.

The other main type of COPD is chronic bronchitis, although both emphysema and chronic bronchitis often occur together. People who suffer from chronic bronchitis have intermittent attacks of obstructed breathing during which their airways become inflamed and clogged with mucus; this often progresses into a condition of continuous obstructed breathing. Historically, chronic bronchitis has occurred more commonly in men than in women, but the condition is becoming more common in women as the prevalence of smoking among women increases.[8]

Asthma

Asthma is characterized by the airway hyperresponsiveness described on page 7. This results in attacks of wheezing, coughing and/or difficulty in breathing.

While smoking doesn't necessarily cause asthma, it does aggravate the condition.[1] Asthmatics who smoke suffer from increased mucus, decreased movement of cilia, increased susceptibility to infection, increased immediate allergic reaction and damage to small airway passages.[9] In one study the rate of death due to asthma among current and former smokers was more than double the death rate due to asthma among nonsmokers. The death rate for people with asthma who had never smoked was 3.7 per 100,000; among current and former smokers it was 8.3 per 100,000.[1]

Respiratory Infections

Smokers suffer more—and more severe—respiratory infections than do nonsmokers. In one study college students who smoked had more coughs, more acute and chronic phlegm production, more wheezing and more lower respiratory tract symptoms with their colds.[10]

Pneumonia is not only more common, but much more likely to be fatal among smokers of any age. Among high-risk or medically compromised adults, the risk of pneumococcal infection is approximately four times as high among those who smoke. Among pregnant women who contract pneumonia, those who smoke more than 10 cigarettes per day are more likely to have an adverse outcome (defined as maternal–fetal death, preterm delivery, fetal death and early miscarriage).[11]

Smoking also makes a person more vulnerable to contracting influenza. In one outbreak of influenza among 336 men in a military unit, 68.5 percent of current and occasional smokers suffered influenza, as compared with 47.2 percent of never and former smokers.[12] Overall, smoking is thought to play a significant role in 31 percent of all influenza cases and 41 percent of severe cases.[11] Vaccination against influenza is less effective in smokers, and the death rate among smokers who suffer influenza is much higher than among nonsmokers.

Finally, in some studies, tuberculosis seems to occur more commonly among smokers; but data are limited.[1]

References

1 Doll R, Peto R, Wheatley K, Gray R, Sutherland I. Papers: Mortality in relation to smoking: 40 years' observations on male British doctors. *Br Med J* 1994;309:901–911.

2 Sherman, CB. The health consequences of cigarette smoking. *Med Clin North Am* 1992;76:355.

3 Hensler NM, Giron DJ. Pulmonary physiological measurements in smokers and nonsmokers *JAMA* 1963;186:885–889.

4 Peterson DI, Lonergan LH, Hardinge MG. Smoking and pulmonary function. *Arch Environ Health* 1968;16:215–218.

5 American Cancer Society. *Cancer Facts and Figures–1996.* 1996.

6 Brownson, RC, Reif JS, Alavanja MCR, Bal DG. Cancer. In: Brownson RC, Remington PL, Davis JR, eds. *Chronic Disease Epidemiology and Control.* Washington, DC: American Public Health Association; 1993.

7 American Lung Association. Chronic obstructive pulmonary disease: emphysema, chronic bronchitis. *Lung Disease Data 1994* 1994; 6–7.

8 Johannsen JM. Chronic obstructive pulmonary disease: current comprehensive care for emphysema and bronchitis. *Nurse Practitioner* 1994;19:59–67.

9 Brook U, Shilow S. Original Articles: Attitudes of asthmatic and nonasthmatic adolescents toward cigarettes and smoking. *Clin Pediatr* 1993;32:642–646.

10 Graham NMH. The epidemiology of acute respiratory infections in children and adults: a global perspective. *Epidemiologic Reviews* 1990;12:159–160.

11 Richey SD. Pneumonia complicating pregnancy. *Obstet Gynecol* 1994;84:525.

12 Blake GH, Abell TD, Stanley WG. Cigarette smoking and upper respiratory infection among recruits in basic combat training. *Ann Intern Med* 1988;109:198–202.

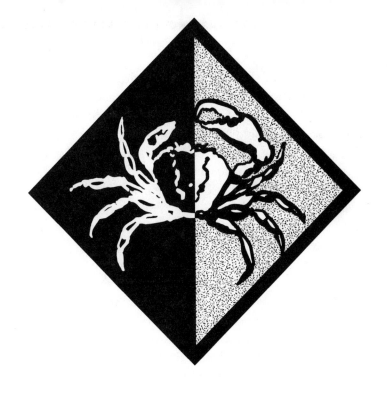

Chapter 2

ONCOLOGY:

SMOKING AND

CANCER RISK

reviewed by
Janet E. Macheledt, M.D., M.S., M.P.H.
Texas Oncology, P.A.
Houston, Texas

Cigarette smoking is the single most important preventable cause of cancer in America today.[1] The American Cancer Society estimated that, in 1995, 170,000 out of 547,000 cancer deaths—nearly one third of all cancer deaths—would be caused by tobacco use. In addition to causing 87 percent of all cases of lung cancer, smoking is associated with cancer at many other sites, including the mouth, pharynx, larynx, esophagus, pancreas, uterine cervix, kidneys, urinary bladder,[2] colon and rectum,[3,4] bone marrow (leukemia) and possibly the stomach. Smokers' overall cancer death rates are twice those of nonsmokers, and the heaviest smokers have overall cancer death rates four times as great as those of nonsmokers.[1] In addition, the percentage of tobacco-linked cancer deaths is increasing, primarily because of the increase in women smokers.

Unlike deaths from many other cancers, the causes of which are not known or are only suspected, cigarette-induced cancer deaths are totally preventable.[2]

In this chapter we will review the association between smoking and cancer, noting, when possible, the relative risk for each type of cancer and the mechanism. (Note, though, that lung cancer was addressed in Chapter 1 and that skin cancer will be covered in Chapter 5.) We also review tenuous tobacco–cancer associations.

Established Associations

While smoking is associated with cancer at many sites, the smoking–cancer connection is especially strong for lung cancer; for head and neck cancers (those involving the esophagus, larynx, tongue, salivary glands, lip, mouth, and pharynx); and for cancers of the urinary bladder, kidney, uterine cervix and pancreas. For certain other cancers, such as colorectal cancer and leukemia, new evidence suggests that smoking may play a role as well.

Head and Neck Cancers

Smoking is the major cause of cancers of the esophagus, larynx, tongue, salivary gland, lip, mouth and pharynx; and the risk increases with the amount and duration of smoking.[5] Tobacco smoking is one of the two strongest determinants for head and neck cancers; alcohol abuse is the other.[6] Consuming alcohol and tobacco together further increases the risk of cancer. Smoking also increases the risk of nasal cancer.

Esophageal cancer. Smoking causes at least 80 percent of all esophageal cancers, claiming 15,000 lives each year from this type of cancer alone.[1] Overall, a smoker's risk of developing esophageal cancer is eight to 10 times greater than that of a nonsmoker. A smoker who abuses alcohol enhances this risk by another 25 to 50 percent.[1]

Experts think smoking causes esophageal cancer by the following mechanism: Although the esophagus is not directly exposed to inhaled cigarette smoke, the constituents of the smoke condense on the mucous membranes of the mouth and pharynx and are then swallowed. The esophagus also receives mucus cleared from the lungs; in cigarette smokers this mucus contains cancer-causing chemicals. It is thought that this continual contact with the chemicals (and their by-products) from cigarette smoke leads to esophageal cancer.[1]

Laryngeal cancer. The risk of laryngeal cancer in heavy smokers is about 12 times greater than the risk in nonsmokers.[6] For all women who smoke, the risk is about eight times greater; for all male smokers, it is about 10 times greater.[1] Smoking is, in fact, the most important cause of laryngeal cancer,[7] accounting for an estimated 82 percent of all cases.[1]

Experts speculate that by-products of various substances in tobacco smoke—especially by-products of aromatic amines and polycyclic aromatic hydrocarbons—are responsible for the toxic changes that induce laryngeal cancer.[7]

Oral cancer. Smoking is the main cause of cancers of the tongue, salivary gland, mouth and pharynx. Approximately 92 percent of oral cancers in men and 61 percent of oral cancers in women are attributable to smoking.[1] Men who smoke are about 27 times more likely to develop oral cancer than men who don't smoke; the increased risk for women smokers is about six times that of nonsmokers.

Some smokers who eventually develop oral cancer first develop a condition called leukoplakia, or white patches in the mouth.[1] Regular dental and mouth examinations can help detect these precancerous lesions, and early therapy can be initiated. Stopping smoking, however, is the only way to avoid cancer.

Nasal cancer. Heavy and long-term smokers have a doubled risk of nasal cancer as compared with nonsmokers.[8]

Bladder and Kidney Cancer

In the Western world, smoking is the strongest risk factor for developing bladder cancer.[9] The 1979 Surgeon General's Report on Smoking concluded that cigarette smoking acts both independently and synergistically (that is, together with other factors) in increasing the risk of bladder cancer.[10] Cigarette smoking accounts for 40 to 70 percent of bladder cancer cases[11] and is responsible for an estimated 7,700[1] bladder cancer deaths yearly. Overall, smokers have a two- to threefold increased risk of bladder cancer as compared with nonsmokers.[12]

Researchers speculate that by-products of the aromatic amines and polycyclic aromatic hydrocarbons found in cigarette smoke are toxic to the lining of the bladder and so induce cancer.[7,11]

Smokers also have an increased risk of kidney cancer. Some estimates put their increased risk as high as five times that of nonsmokers, with risk increasing as the amount smoked increases.[10]

Pancreatic Cancer

It is estimated that 30 percent of the 8,000 yearly deaths from pancreatic cancer[1] are due to smoking. Overall, a smoker has about twice the risk of a nonsmoker of developing pancreatic cancer; someone who smokes more than 40 cigarettes per day has about a fivefold increase in risk.[1]

The most likely explanation of how smoking causes pancreatic cancer is that the cancer-causing substances in cigarette smoke—and their by-products—reach the tissues of the pancreas via the blood and bile (bile is fluid released by the liver and discharged into the small intestine to aid in digestion).[1]

Leukemia

Leukemia is the term used to refer to a variety of white blood cell cancers that arise from bone marrow. Increasing evidence suggests that cigarette smoking causes some forms of adult leukemia.[13]

Genital Cancer

A study of the association between smoking and genital cancer (including, but not limited to, vulvular, cervical and penile cancer) found that smokers had an increased risk at all sites but that the risks were especially great with vulvular and penile cancers.[14] The immunosuppressive effects of smoking cigarettes and the carcinogenic action of cigarette smoke acting either directly (on the skin) or indirectly (through exposure via body fluids) are plausible reasons for the increase in the risk of these cancers among smokers.[15]

Vulvular cancer: Cancer of the vulva, part of the female genitalia, is quite rare; the annual incidence rate is just 1.6 per 100,000 women. Women who smoke double their risk of developing this type of cancer, and the risk becomes even greater with heavier smoking.[16,17] Experts theorize that smoking-induced abnormalities in the immune system may play a role.[16]

Cervical cancer: The association of smoking with cervical cancer has been recognized only recently; the Centers for Disease Control and Prevention added cervical cancer to the categories of smoking-induced disease in 1988.[18] While smokers as a group commonly have other risk factors associated with cervical cancer (including multiple sexual partners and the presence of sexually transmitted diseases), at least 12 studies have found that smoking increases the risk for cervical cancer after accounting for these other factors.[10] Approximately 1,400[1] cervical cancer deaths each year (about 31 percent of the 4,514 total deaths) are estimated to be due to smoking.

Cervical cancer risk increases with both the time and the amount smoked; by some estimates, women who smoke more than 40 cigarettes per day increase their risk about two and a half times over that of non-smokers.[19]

Smoking may increase cervical cancer by one or more mechanisms. It is possible, for example, that nicotine exerts some direct effect on the tissues of the cervix. Studies have shown that nicotine can be found in these tissues.[19] It is also possible that smoking enhances the effect of other factors known to increase the risk of cervical cancer. The human papilloma virus has recently been shown to be responsible for the majority of cervical cancer diagnosed today. Some investigators hypothesize that smoking makes the virus an even stronger cancer-causing agent.[20] Another theory is that smokers' cancer risk is higher because smoking makes the immune system weaker[21] and less able to fight the cancer-causing infections.

Penile cancer: One study has estimated more than a doubling of penile cancer risk among men who smoke more than 10 cigarettes per day as compared with nonsmokers.[22] Another study has estimated more than a tripling of risk for people with a history of more than 45 pack-years.[23]

Anal and Colorectal Cancer

Anal cancer: One study has estimated that the risk of anal cancer is elevated by almost eight times for heterosexual men who smoke and by more than nine times for women who smoke.[24]

Colorectal cancer: As in the case of cervical cancer, there is relatively recent evidence that smoking plays some role in colorectal cancer. Early studies found little or no increased risk of colorectal cancer among smokers[25,26]; but two recent studies, one of men and one of women, suggest that cigarette smoking induces colon cancer and its precursor adenomas (often called polyps) in both men and women.[3,4]

The 47,935 men studied are part of the ongoing Health Professionals Follow-up Study; the 118,334 women are part of the ongoing Nurses' Health Study. Smoking (measured in total lifetime pack-years) was associated in both men and women with an increased risk of small polyps, large polyps and cancer. Further, in both men and women the risk increased with the amount smoked. Overall, both men and women who smoked had a 75- to 100-percent increased risk of developing colorectal cancer as compared with their nonsmoking peers. Unfortunately, the enhanced cancer risk doesn't return to normal when the smoker gives up the habit; the increased risk remains for the rest of an ex-smoker's lifetime.

In addition, the type of abnormality—small polyp, large polyp or cancer—was dependent on the length of time a person smoked. Smoking in the previous 20 years was associated with the prevalence of small polyps. Smoking in the previous 20 to 35 years was associated with the risk of large polyps. Finally, cigarette smoking more than 35 years in the past was associated with colon cancer.

These results show that in the case of colorectal cancer there may be an induction period, or lag time, of up to 35 years for the cancer to develop. This is important for two reasons. First, with a long induction period, there might be considerable benefit to be gained from early and regular screening, since polyps caught early can be removed, thereby preventing cancer from forming. Second, this long induction period from the onset of smoking to the development of cancer might explain why it was difficult to establish this relationship in earlier studies.[27]

Finally, another study, this one of U.S. veterans, showed significant increases in colon cancer among cigarette smokers. Among 248,046 veterans studied for 26 years, colon cancer mortality increased with pack-years of smoking.[28]

Tenuous Associations
Smoking and Breast Cancer
Many investigators have studied the relationship of smoking to breast cancer, but with conflicting results. At least four studies have found that smoking decreased breast cancer risk, possibly by reducing the amount of estrogen in a woman's body. Three studies have found that smoking increased the risk of breast cancer. And at least nine studies have reported absolutely no association.[29] One study in which women who had smoked in their teens were compared with women who had never smoked found that smoking during adolescence doubled the risk of breast cancer later in life.[30]

A recent report suggested that women with breast cancer who had smoked over 10,000 packs in a lifetime had a risk of the cancer spreading to the lungs that was over three times higher than the risk of nonsmokers.[31] Smoking has also been shown to predict fatal breast cancer in a dose-response relationship: Smokers of 40 or more cigarettes a day have almost twice the rate of fatal breast cancers as nonsmokers. This increased risk may, however, be attributable to smokers' being less likely than nonsmokers to get mammograms rather than to the effects of smoking.[32]

It appears at this point that the evidence does not consistently show that smoking plays a role in the development of breast cancer.

Smoking and Prostate Cancer
There is an abundance of literature on smoking and prostate cancer, most of which does not support an association. Only three studies have reported that smoking appeared to be related to the development of prostate cancer, while 20 studies found no association.[33] However, even though smoking has not been shown to be responsible for the development of prostate cancer, smokers may be at a greater risk for more aggressive disease, or cancer that advances more rapidly. One study found that smokers had a higher incidence of more invasive and high-grade prostate cancer than did nonsmokers.[34] In addition, smokers with prostate cancer are more likely to die from their cancer than are nonsmokers with the same disease.[35,36]

One explanation for this is that smoking reduces blood flow to the prostate gland through vasoconstriction (continued or chronic constriction of the blood vessels), which may make the gland more susceptible to the toxic effects of the potentially cancerous compounds in cigarette smoke—especially tar, nicotine and the aromatic amines (such as benzopyrene). These compounds may induce a more aggressive, highly invasive type of cancer.

Stomach Cancer

Smokers appear to have a modest increase in their risk of stomach cancer—just 50 percent over the risk of nonsmokers. If this association is causal, then at least one fifth of stomach cancer would be attributable to smoking.[1]

References

1 Newcomb PA, Carbone PP. The health consequences of smoking: cancer. *Med Clin North Am* 1992;76:305–331.

2 American Cancer Society. *Cancer Facts and Figures—1995*.

3 Giovannucci E, Rimm EB, Stampfer MJ, et al. A prospective study of cigarette smoking and risk of colorectal adenoma and colorectal cancer in U.S. men. *JNCI* 1994;86:183–191.

4 Giovannucci E, Colditz GA, Stampfer MJ. A prospective study of cigarette smoking and risk of colorectal adenoma and colorectal cancer in U.S. women. *JNCI* 1994;86:192–199.

5 Tuyns AJ. Ætiology of head and neck cancer: tobacco, alcohol and diet. *Otolaryngology* 1991;46:98–106.

6 Maier H, Dietz A, Gewelke U, et al. Tobacco and alcohol and the risk of head and neck cancer. *Clinical Investigator* 1992;70:320–327.

7 Lafuente A, Pujol F, Carretero P, et al. Human glutathione S-transferase m(GSTm) deficiency as a marker for the susceptibility to bladder and larynx cancer among smokers. *Cancer Letters* 1993;68:49–54.

8 Zheng W, McLaughlin JK, Chow WH, et al. Risk factors for cancers of the nasal cavity and paranasal sinuses among white men in the United States. *Am J Epidemiol* 1993;138:965–972.

9 Salminen E, Pukkala E, Teppo L. Bladder cancer and the risk of smoking-related cancers during followup. *J Urology* 1994;152:1420–1423.

10 *Reducing the Health Consequences of Smoking: 25 Years of Progress. A Report of the Surgeon General.* Rockville, MD: US Department of Health and Human Services, Centers for Disease Control; 1989:56.

11 Talaska G, Schamer M, Casetta G, et al. Carcinogen-DNA adducts in bladder biopsies and urothelial cells: a risk assessment exercise. *Cancer Letters* 1994;84:93–97.

12 Spruck CH, Rideout WM, Olumi AR. Distinct pattern of p53 mutations in bladder cancer: relationship to tobacco usage. *Cancer Research* 1993;53:1162–1166.

13 Brownson R, Novotny TE, Perry MC. Cigarette smoking and adult leukemia: a meta-analysis. *Arch Intern Med* 1993; 153:469–475.

14 Daling JR, Sherman KJ, Hislop TG, et al. Cigarette smoking and the risk of anogenital cancer. *Am J Epidemiol* 1992; 135:180–189. Cited in Smith JB, Fenske NA. Cutaneous manifestations and consequences of smoking. *J Am Acad Dermatol* 1996; 34:717–732.

15 Smith JB, Fenske NA. Cutaneous manifestations and consequences of smoking. *J Am Acad Dermatol* 1996; 34:717–732.

16 Brinton LA, Nasca PC, Malliln K. Case-control study of cancer of the vulva. *Obstet Gynecol* 1990;75:859.

17 Newcomb PA, Weiss NS, Daling JR. Incidence of vulvar carcinoma in relation to menstrual, reproductive and medical factors. *JNCI* 1984;391–396.

18 Lipsitz CM. Have you come a long way, baby? Smoking trends in women. *Maryland Medical Journal* 1993;42:27–31.

19 Brinton LA. Editorial commentary: smoking and cervical cancer—current status. *Am J Epidemiol* 1990;131:958–960.

20 Herrero R, Brinton LA, Reeves WC, et al. Invasive cervical cancer and smoking in Latin America. *JNCI* 1989;81:205–211.

21 Barton SE, Jenkins D, Cuzick J, et al. Effect of cigarette smoking on cervical epithelial immunity: a mechanism for neoplastic change? *Lancet* 1988:2:652–654.

22 Hellberg D, Valentin J, Eklund T, et al. Penile cancer: is there an epidemiological role for smoking and sexual behavior? *Br Med J* 1987;295:1306–1308. Cited in Smith JB, Fenske NA. Cutaneous manifestations and consequences of smoking. *J Am Acad Dermatol* 1996; 34:717–732.

23 Maden C, Sherman KJ, Beckmann AM. History of circumcision, medical conditions, and sexual activity and risk of penile cancer. *J Natl Cancer Inst* 1993:85:19–24. Cited in Smith JB, Fenske NA. Cutaneous manifestations and consequences of smoking. *J Am Acad Dermatol* 1996; 34:717–732.

24 Daling JR, Weiss NS, Hislop G, et al. Sexual practices, sexually transmitted diseases, and the incidence of anal cancer. *N Engl J Med* 1987;317:973–977. Cited in Smith JB, Fenske NA. Cutaneous manifestations and consequences of smoking. *J Am Acad Dermatol* 1996; 34:717–732.

25 Slattery ML, West DW, Robison LM, et al. Tobacco, alcohol, coffee, and caffeine as risk factors for colon cancer in a low risk population. *Epidemiology* 1990;1:141–145.

26 Chute CG, Willett WC, Colditz GA, et al. A prospective study of body mass, height, and smoking on the risk of colorectal cancer in women. *Cancer Causes and Control* 1991;2:117–124.

27 Fielding JE. Editorial: preventing colon cancer: yet another reason not to smoke. *JNCI* 1994;86:162.

28 Heineman EF, Zahm SH, McLaughlin JK, Vaught JB. Increased risk of colorectal cancer among smokers: results of a 26-year follow-up of US veterans and a review. *Int J Cancer* 1994; 59(6):728–738.

29 Chu SY, Stroup NE, Wingo PA. Cigarette smoking and the risk of breast cancer. *Am J Epidemiol* 1990;131:244–253.

30 Palmer JR, Rosenberg L, Clarke A, et al. Breast cancer and cigarette smoking: a hypothesis. *Am J Epidemiol* 1991;134:1–13.

31 Scanlon EF, Suh O, Murthy SM, Mettlin C, Reid SE, Cummings KM. Influence of smoking on the development of lung metastases from breast cancer. *Cancer* 1995;75:2693–2699.

32 Calle EE, Miracle-McMahill HL, Thun MJ, Heath, Jr., CW. Cigarette smoking and risk of fatal breast cancer. *Am J Epidemiol* 1994;139:1001–1007.

33 van der Gulden JWJ, Verbeek ALM, Kolk JJ. Smoking and drinking habits in relation to prostate cancer. *Br J Urology* 1994;73:382–389.

34 Hussain F, Aziz H, Macchia R. High grade adenocarcinoma of prostate in smokers of ethnic minority groups and Caribbean island immigrants. *J Radiation Oncology Biol Phys* 1992;24:451–461.

35 Hsing AW, McLaughlin JK, Hrubec Z, et al. Tobacco use and prostate cancer: 26-year follow-up of veterans. *Am J Epidemiol* 1991;133:437.

36 Hsing AW, McLaughlin JK, Schuman LM, et al. Diet, tobacco use and fatal prostate cancer: results from the Lutheran Brotherhood Cohort Study. *Cancer Res* 1990;50:6836.

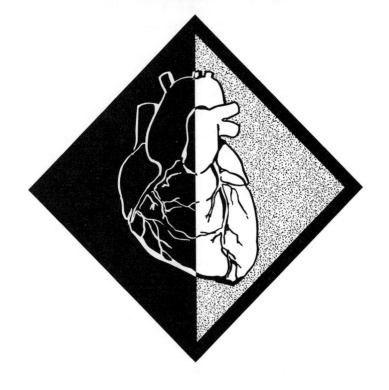

Chapter 3

SMOKING

AND HEART

DISEASE

reviewed by
Eric Topol, M.D.
Chairman, Division of Cardiology
The Cleveland Clinic
Foundation

Each year, cigarette smoking accounts for nearly 200,000, or one fifth, of all deaths from heart disease in the United States.[1] Since 1940, when researchers at the Mayo Clinic in Rochester, Minnesota, linked cigarette smoking to an elevated risk for heart disease (also called cardiovascular disease), mounting evidence has provided overwhelming evidence that smoking increases a person's risk of developing several types of heart disease. And despite popular belief to the contrary, smoking even a few cigarettes per day raises the risk.[2] In a recent study of female nurses, women who smoked just one to four cigarettes per day had a 2.5-fold increased risk of fatal coronary heart disease.[1]

Included among the heart diseases for which smokers are at higher risk are atherosclerosis, coronary heart disease, stroke, angina, irregular heart beats, sudden death, heart attack, fatal heart attack and aortic aneurysm.[1] Of these, coronary heart disease (CHD) is the most important, accounting for over half of the heart-disease deaths caused by smoking. According to the Centers for Disease Control and Prevention (CDC), the estimated number of preventable deaths in the United States each year from CHD related to smoking is over 90,000.[3] The U.S. Surgeon General has called cigarette smoking "the most important of the known modifiable risk factors for CHD."[4] It is thought that another 37,000 deaths from atherosclerosis are caused by passive smoking each year,[5] but those data—unlike those for smokers themselves—are speculative. In addition, smoking raises blood pressure, which also contributes to heart disease risk.[6]

In this chapter, we look at the immediate effects of smoking on the heart and blood vessels and then review the types of heart disease caused by smoking.

How Smoking Affects the Heart and its Blood Vessels

Inhaling tobacco smoke causes several immediate responses within the heart and its blood vessels. One major response that a smoker might notice after smoking is an increase in heart rate. This may be the only perceived response, but as a stimulant to the autonomic nervous system—the part of the nervous system that controls involuntary functions—smoking causes several other changes that affect the heart. Within one minute of starting to smoke, the heart rate begins to rise; it may increase by as much as 30 percent during the first 10 minutes of smoking. The heart rate may decrease slightly as smoking continues, but it does not return to normal until after smoking has stopped.[2]

The other important response to this stimulation is an acute increase in blood pressure. The blood vessels constrict, or clamp down, which forces the heart to work harder to try to deliver oxygen to the rest of the body and to the heart muscle itself.

Another ingredient of tobacco smoke, carbon monoxide, exerts a powerful negative effect on the heart by compromising the blood's ability to carry oxygen.

Hypertension

While some studies suggest that blood pressure returns to normal between episodes of smoking, repeated smoking throughout the day results in higher average pressures. Smoking also results in greater blood pressure variability, or swings in blood pressure. While hypertension itself can lead to heart disease, variable hypertension is even more dangerous and even more likely to lead to heart damage.[2]

Smoking also reduces the effectiveness of treatment for high blood pressure. Some studies indicate that smoking actually neutralizes hypertension medication. One way in which it might do this is by causing the liver to release into the bloodstream enzymes that render blood pressure medications less effective.[6]

Coronary Heart Disease

The leading cause of coronary heart disease is atherosclerosis, a clogging and narrowing of the arteries that supply blood to the heart muscle. The arteries become narrower after their lining is damaged because fatty substances and fibrous tissues collect along the damaged inner lining. The lining can become damaged through a number of factors: high blood pressure, toxic chemicals (such as those found in cigarette smoke) and a high concentration of blood fats.

The damaged arteries become an attractive site for blood fats and platelets (a clotting factor in the blood) to accumulate. Once the blood fats and platelets have begun to accumulate, the area becomes a catch-all for cell debris and cholesterol. Finally, the formation of scarlike tissue gives rise to an atherosclerotic plaque. The same chemicals (e.g., polycyclic aro-

vasoconstriction

27

matic hydrocarbons) that are implicated in smoking-induced cancers also appear to have atherogenic (plaque-forming) activity.

Although most smokers don't realize it, smoking is just as potent a risk factor for developing atherosclerosis as are high blood pressure (hypertension) and high blood cholesterol.[6] In combination with these other risk factors, smoking exerts a tremendously powerful effect, creating a risk far greater than what would be expected just from adding the two risks together. This is what is known as a synergistic effect—a multiplying of risk factors that occur together.[6] Overall, smokers have a two- to fourfold greater incidence of CHD and about a 70 percent greater death rate from it.[7]

There are several reasons smoking leads to atherosclerosis. Over time, the continued or chronic constriction of the blood vessels (vasoconstriction) that occurs in response to smoking causes the interior of the vessels to become damaged. The damaged blood vessels, in turn, are more susceptible to accumulating plaque. And once plaque is present in the vessels, smoking encourages the progression of the artery-clogging process. The chronic vasoconstriction also causes blood clots to form on the plaque lesions. When the plaque itself becomes damaged during vasoconstriction, the lining of the blood vessels and the platelets both release additional substances; that, in turn, leads to even greater vasoconstriction. A cycle begins that can lead to formation of clots, blockage of arteries and finally a heart attack.

In addition to causing vasoconstriction, smoking leads to atherosclerosis by causing abnormalities in the blood components that affect clotting, both those that promote clotting and those that keep it in check. Smoking directly reduces the life span of platelets and causes them to clump together abnormally. Independent of that, smoking causes the platelets to be stickier than normal, again causing them to be more likely to clump. That clumping in turn leads to blood-clot formation, which is compounded by smoking's effects on the blood's anticlotting factors. Smoking hinders factors that dissolve tiny blood clots which continually form in the bloodstream.

Doctors often prescribe aspirin for people at high risk of heart disease because the aspirin helps prevent the clot formation that can lead to heart disease. In smokers, however, aspirin is less effective for controlling clot formation.

Additionally, smoking causes clogged arteries by the multiple effects it has on blood fats, or blood lipids. The nicotine exposure resulting from smoking causes higher levels of free fatty acids in the bloodstream. In particular, this exposure causes higher levels of very low density lipoproteins (VLDL), a type of blood fat that negatively impacts other types of blood fats. VLDL raises levels of LDL-cholesterol, the bad cholesterol, and decreases levels of HDL, or good, cholesterol.

Smoking interferes with the normal metabolism of cholesterol and triglycerides. In particular, smoking has two negative effects on HDL-cholesterol. Not only does smoking reduce the (good) HDL-cholesterol, but it also changes the composition of the remaining HDL-cholesterol, rendering it less able to exert its antiatherogenic (anti–artery-clogging) effects. And smoking's negative effect on HDL-cholesterol increases with the number of cigarettes smoked per day.

In women, smoking is also associated with an earlier menopause. The onset of menopause raises heart-disease risk because postmenopausal women produce much less estrogen, a hormone known to protect against heart disease. Even female smokers who have not yet reached menopause have estrogen levels that are lower than normal, a factor that increases their heart-disease risk. Postmenopausal smokers who undergo estrogen replacement therapy do not achieve as high a level of blood estrogen as do nonsmokers.[6] Smoking "induces" enzymes from the liver to break down estrogen at a faster rate than occurs in nonsmokers.

While medical advances have led to very effective therapies to clear clogged arteries, these therapies are less effective over the long run in smokers. Smokers who continue to smoke after angioplasty, for example, are more likely to experience recurrence of their disease and to require a repeat angioplasty than are nonsmokers.[8]

Angina and Heart Attack

If an artery or arteries in the heart go into spasm, blood supply to the heart is reduced. The immediate symptom of this condition, called ischemia, is chest pain, or angina. If the heart muscle doesn't receive adequate oxygen for a long enough period of time, part of the muscle actually dies. This is generally known as a "heart attack." Smokers experience both more angina and more heart attacks than do nonsmokers. The evidence is strong that first heart attacks occur earlier in smokers than in nonsmokers.[9,10]

When compared with people who have never smoked, smokers have over 20 times the risk of developing angina.[6] Beyond the typical exercise-induced angina, smoking is also a major risk factor for vasospastic angina (chest pain occurring at rest due to spasm of the coronary arteries).[11] Remarkably, spasm of the coronary arteries can occur after smoking just one cigarette.[6]

Smokers experience more angina and suffer angina attacks at much lower activity levels than nonsmokers. In addition, medications used to treat angina are less effective in smokers. In one study smokers with heart disease experienced 33 percent more episodes of ischemia per day than did nonsmokers with heart disease—and the smokers' ischemic events lasted longer.[12]

As mentioned above, plaque that becomes damaged by continued smoking and vasoconstriction can release clots that can lodge in the heart and block blood flow to part of the heart muscle. This blood flow is compromised by two additional mechanisms: the rises in heart rate and in blood pressure that occur in response to smoking.

Because the heart is working harder to supply oxygen to the body under less than optimal conditions, it requires more and more oxygen itself. At the same time, in the presence of cigarette smoke, the vessels that supply blood to the heart are less able to regulate the flow of blood to the heart muscle. This means that despite the fact that the heart is "asking" for more oxygen, it cannot get it because of the adverse conditions. Smoking even a single cigarette can result in a significant decrease in blood flow to an entire section of the heart.[6]

The carbon monoxide in cigarette smoke (it makes up from 2.7 to 6 percent of the smoke) also reduces the oxygen-carrying capacity of the blood. Cigarette smoke averages about 400 parts per million of carbon monoxide—eight times greater than the maximum level of carbon monoxide permitted in industry.[13]

All of these insults taken together significantly compromise the health of the heart muscle.

In addition to suffering more heart attacks, smokers are more likely to suffer *repeat* heart attacks. According to one estimate, cigarette smoking increases the risk in one year for a recurrent heart attack from a nonsmoker's 6.3 percent to 12.5 percent.[6]

Some smokers mistakenly believe that smoking cigarettes that are lower in tar and nicotine reduces their risk of heart disease. Ads for such cigarettes target smokers who are concerned about the health effects of their dangerous habit. But research has now demonstrated that these so-called "lower yield" cigarettes do not provide any reduction in risk for a first nonfatal heart attack.[14]

Arrhythmia (Irregular Heartbeat) and Sudden Death

Smoking causes an increased release of catecholamines, natural body chemicals such as adrenaline that ultimately can interfere with the heart's normal rhythm. This interference can cause arrhythmias, or abnormal heart rhythms. In particular, smokers have much higher rates than non-smokers of two potentially serious arrhythmias: the deadly arrhythmia called ventricular fibrillation and ventricular premature beats. Arrhythmias are potentially dangerous when they occur in isolation, but they also increase the sufferer's chances of dying of a heart attack.

Aortic Aneurysm

The aorta is the large artery carrying oxygenated blood from the heart to the rest of the body. Anyone can develop atherosclerosis in the aorta, but smokers have an exceptionally high risk of developing extensive atherosclerosis there. Atherosclerosis within the aorta can cause it to weaken and develop an aneurysm, or an outpouching of the vessel wall. Such a weakened vessel wall may rupture. Smokers have about eight times the risk of aortic aneurysms—and much higher death rates from ruptured aortic aneurysms—than do nonsmokers.[15]

Cardiomyopathy

Cardiomyopathy is a disease that leads to extensive, progressive damage to the heart muscle, resulting in severe fatigue and shortness of breath. Over time, the heart loses its ability to function and maintain life. A heart transplant may then become necessary.

Accumulating evidence now indicates that the risk of developing cardiomyopathy is much greater in smokers. Smoking may bring on the disease by damaging small arteries, or perhaps the carbon monoxide in cigarette smoke damages the heart muscle directly. It's also possible that smoking increases the heart muscle's susceptibility to a viral infection that in turn leads to cardiomyopathy.[16]

Stop Now—It Does Make a Difference

Stopping smoking does make a difference. According to the Framingham Heart Study, relatively light smokers (those who smoke 10 cigarettes per day) have a 20 percent reduction of their heart attack risk two years after quitting. Heavy smokers (those who smoke more than 40 cigarettes per day) realize significant gains—an almost 60 percent reduction of their heart attack risk.[6]

Stopping smoking also slashes a person's risk of dying from a ruptured aortic aneurysm by approximately 50 percent. A former smoker, however, still has a two- to three-times greater risk of dying from an aortic aneurysm than does someone who has never smoked.[6]

From 1988 to 1990 there was a 10.4 percent decline in deaths in the United States from cardiovascular disease.[1] An estimated 24 percent of this overall decline was related to the reduction in cigarette smoking.[6] Unfortunately, the prevalence of smoking among U.S. adults did not decline between 1990 and 1991.[1]

References

1   Bartecchi CE, et al. *N Engl J Med* 1994;330:907–912.

2   DeCasaris R, Ranieri G, Filitti V, et al. Cardiovascular effects of cigarette smoking. *Cardiology* 1992;81:236.

3   As cited in McBride PE. *Med Clin North Am* 1992;76:333–353.

4   US Department of Health and Human Services. *The Health Benefits of Smoking Cessation—a report of the Surgeon General* 1990; page 197.

5   Glantz SA, Parmley WW. Passive smoking and heart disease: Epidemiology, physiology and biochemistry. *Circulation* 1991; 83:1–12.

6   McBride PE. *Med Clin North Am* 1992;76:333–353.

7   US Department of Health and Human Services. *Reducing the Health Consequences of Smoking—25 Years of Progress. A Report of the Surgeon General.* U.S. Department of Health and Human Services, Public Health Service, Office on Smoking and Health, 1989.

8   Galan KM, Deligonul U, Kern MJ, et al: Increased frequency of restenosis in patients continuing to smoke cigarettes after percutaneous transluminal coronary angioplasty. *Am J Cardiol* 1988;61:260–263.

9   Gottlieb S, Fallavollita J, McDermott M, Brown M, Eberly S, Moss AJ. Cigarette smoking and the age of onset of a first non-fatal myocardial infarction. *Coron Artery Dis* 1994;5:687–694.

10 Parish S, Collins R, Peto R, et al. Cigarette smoking, tar yields, and non-fatal myocardial infarction: 14,000 cases and 32,000 controls in the United Kingdom. The International Studies of Infarct Survival (ISIS) Collaborators. *Br Med J* 1995;311:471–477.

11 Sugiishi M. Coronary circulation: cigarette smoking is a major risk factor for coronary spasm. *Circulation* 1993;87:76–79.

12 Barry J, Mead K, Nabel EG, et al. Effect of smoking on the activity of ischemic heart disease. *JAMA* 1989;261:398–402.

13 Turino GM. Effect of carbon monoxide on the cardiorespiratory system. Carbon monoxide toxicity: physiology and biochemistry. *Circulation* 1981;63(1):253A–259A.

14 Palmer JR, Rosenberg L, Shapiro S. 'Low yield' cigarettes: the risk of nonfatal myocardial infarction in women. *N Engl J Med* 1989;320:1569–1573.

15 Auerbach D, Garfinkel L. Atherosclerosis and aneurysm of the aorta in relation to smoking habits and age. *Chest* 78:805–809.

16 Hartz AJ, Anderson AJ, Brooks HL, et al. The association of smoking with cardiomyopathy. *N Engl J Med* 1984;311:1201–1206.

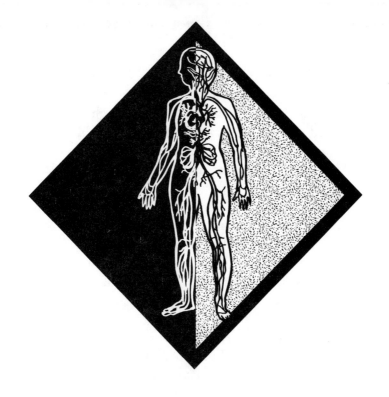

Chapter 4

SMOKING

AND PERIPHERAL

VASCULAR

DISEASE

reviewed by
Carmen Fonseca, M.D.
Department of Vascular Medicine
The Cleveland Clinic
Foundation

There is no question that smoking injures the blood vessels of the heart. The damage, however, is not limited to blood vessels there; smoking also causes serious damage to blood vessels throughout the body. Damage to blood vessels in the brain leads to strokes, which can cause permanent brain damage. Chapter 12 addresses smoking and strokes; this chapter will address peripheral vascular occlusive disease, or blocked blood vessels in the legs and feet.

Current smokers have a risk of developing peripheral vascular disease 16 times greater than that of people who have never smoked. Former smokers are seven times more likely to develop the disorder than are those who have never smoked.[1] In fact, smoking accounts for about 76 percent of all peripheral vascular disease.[1] It overshadows all other major risk factors, including diabetes, obesity, hypertension, blood-fat abnormalities and blood-clotting disorders.[2]

Peripheral vascular disease can have consequences that are painful, disabling and even life threatening. In addition, people who continue to smoke after being treated for the disease are far less likely to be treated successfully.[3]

This chapter will first describe why blood vessels are damaged by smoking and then go on to describe peripheral vascular disease in greater detail.

How Blood Vessels are Damaged

There are several mechanisms by which peripheral blood vessels (vessels in the outlying parts of the body, such as the legs and feet) are damaged by smoking:

Peripheral resistance: Smoking decreases blood flow to the extremities by a phenomenon called peripheral resistance.[4] Peripheral resistance is caused by the smoking-induced release of catecholamines. These naturally occurring chemicals increase heart rate, raise blood pressure and cause the blood vessels to constrict.[5] In one study smoking a single cigarette reduced digital blood-flow velocity (the speed at which blood flows through the vessels in the fingers) by approximately 50 percent for at least 30 to 50 minutes.[6] The decreased blood flow deprives these vessels of oxygen and vital nutrients, and that deprivation leads to damage.

Platelet clumping (platelet aggregation): Platelets are one of the components in the bloodstream that cause blood to clot in response to bleeding. Through many chemical controls, the body maintains just the right amount of platelet clumping—not too much and not too little. But external factors such as cigarette smoke can cause platelet clumping to go awry, making blood clot too much.[7] Too much platelet clumping can wear on blood vessels, damaging them.[5]

Smoking disables at least one mechanism by which the body controls platelet clumping—prostaglandins. While normal levels of prostaglandins help blood to clot normally, unchecked levels can cause platelets to clump excessively, which is what happens when smoking disables the prostaglandins.

There are at least two other mechanisms by which smoking causes platelets to clump too much. First, at least one ingredient of tobacco smoke, carbon monoxide, combines with hemoglobin to form carboxyhemoglobin, which causes platelets to aggregate. Second, the nicotine in tobacco smoke also contributes to platelet aggregation.[3] Smoking-induced changes in platelet function persist for at least a week after the last cigarette is smoked.[8]

Increased levels of another blood clotting factor: Levels of fibrinogen, another factor in the blood necessary for normal blood clotting, are abnormally increased in smokers. A smoker's body also loses part of its normal ability to break down fibrinogen levels.[3] This creates yet another mechanism by which blood clots too much and subsequently damages blood vessels.

Damaged blood-vessel lining: Some components of cigarette smoke directly attack and damage the lining of blood vessels, causing small tears.[3,7] Damaged blood vessels are much more likely to attract blood fats and other substances that attach to and then block blood vessels.

Altered red blood cell shape: Smoking makes red blood cells more rigid and less pliable. Altered red blood cells do not flow through the blood vessels as easily; they thus impair blood flow and further damage blood vessels.[3]

Increased "thickness" of blood: Smoking also increases blood viscosity, making the blood thicker.[3] Although results aren't entirely consistent, some studies have shown that at least part of this greater viscosity is due to significantly higher hemoglobin levels in smokers. The hemoglobin levels may be higher in smokers' blood to compensate for the carboxyhemoglobin that forms there[2] from the carbon monoxide in cigarette smoke. This thicker blood is more apt to damage blood vessels.

What Happens in Peripheral Vascular Disease

Peripheral vascular disease develops silently; very often, people don't know they're affected until they experience pain when they walk. They stop until the pain subsides and then start walking again. This repeating cycle is called intermittent claudication and is a sign of extensive disease. As the disease progresses, its victims experience this disabling pain even at rest.

But people with intermittent claudication do not simply have seriously impaired blood flow to their legs and feet; they also are at greater risk of death. The mortality among patients with this disorder is two to three times greater than that of the general population.[1]

In the later stages of peripheral vascular disease, open sores develop in the legs and feet. These sores can progress to gangrene, or the death of affected tissue.[9] About 5 percent of the people who develop this serious form of peripheral vascular disease eventually must undergo amputation.[1] Smokers undergoing amputation for severe peripheral vascular disease are, on average, 6.4 years younger than nonsmokers who must have a limb amputated. In addition, smokers' risk of reinfection and further amputation is at least two and a half times as great.[5]

Smoking also increases the risk of *thromboangiitis obliterans,* or Buerger's disease, an inflammatory condition of small vessels that leads to arterial occlusion and gangrene, first of the toes and then of the foot.

References

1 Cole CW, Farzad E, Bouchard A, et al. Cigarette smoking and peripheral arterial occlusive disease. *Surgery* 1993;114:753–757.

2 Castleden WM, Faulkner K, House AK, Watt A. Hæmoglobin, smoking and peripheral vascular disease. *J Royal Soc Med* 1981;74:586.

3 Belch JJF, McArdle BM, Burns P. The effects of acute smoking on platelet behaviour, fibrinolysis and hæmorheology in habitual smokers. *Thromb Haemostas* (Stuttgart 1984;51:6–8).

4 McBride PE. *Med Clin North Am* 1992;76:339.

5 Lind J, Kramhoft M, Bodtker S. The influence of smoking on complications after primary amputations of the lower extremity. *Clin Orthop* 1991;267:211–217.

6 Sarin CL, Austin JC, Nickel WO. Effects of smoking on digital blood-flow velocity. *JAMA* 1974;229:1327.

7 Davis J, Shelton, L. Effects of tobacco and non-tobacco cigarette smoking on endothelium and platelets. *Clin Pharmacol Ther* 1985;37:529–533.

8 Nowak J, Murray JJ, Oates JA, Fitzgerald GA. Biochemical evidence of a chronic abnormality in platelet and vascular function in healthy individuals who smoke cigarettes. *Circulation* 1987;86:6.

9 Vogt MT, Cauley JA, Kuller LH, Hulley SB. Prevalence and correlates of lower extremity arterial disease in elderly women. *Am J Epidemiol* 1993;137:559–568.

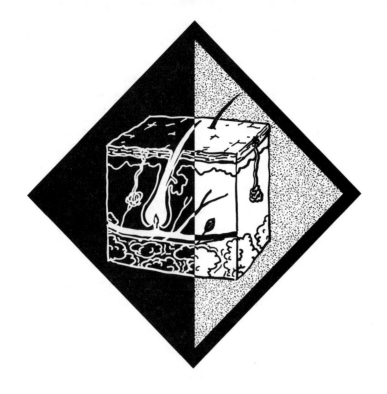

Chapter 5

SMOKING

AND THE SKIN

reviewed by Wilma F. Bergfeld, M.D.
The Cleveland Clinic Foundation
Past President,
American Academy
of Dermatologists

If you were to line up 10 middle-aged smokers on one side of a room and 10 nonsmokers of similar age on the other, chances are you would notice one striking difference: The smokers would look much older than the nonsmokers. The reason? The skin of middle-aged smokers is substantially more wrinkled. Smokers in their 40s have facial wrinkles similar to those of nonsmokers in their 60s.[1]

Another telltale sign of cigarette smoking is a yellow-brown discoloration of the fingernails, usually of the fingers that hold cigarettes.[2]

Smoking is also a risk factor for a skin condition more serious than wrinkles or fingernail discoloration: psoriasis. In this chapter we'll discuss how the changes smoking causes in the skin can lead to wrinkles and psoriasis. Smoking will also be discussed in relation to skin cancer. Finally, we'll also touch on a study suggesting an apparent decrease in risk for acne among smokers.

How Smoking Affects the Skin

The skin is affected by smoke in at least two major ways. First, the by-products of smoke released into the environment—secondhand or environmental tobacco smoke—are an immediate and direct irritant to the skin's surface, possibly exerting a drying effect.[3] Second, because smoking constricts blood vessels, it ultimately reduces the amount of blood—and the nutrients blood contains—flowing to the skin.[4,5,6,7] Some research suggests that smoking may reduce the body's stores of vitamin A, which provides protection against some skin-damaging agents produced by smoking.[8] Another reasonable speculation is that squinting in response to the irritating nature of tobacco smoke on the eyes may contribute to wrinkling.[9]

According to some researchers, the damage to a smoker's skin is analogous to the damage inflicted on the lungs, which are similarly assaulted by smoking.[9] Skin damaged as a result of smoking has a wasted appearance, a condition known as atrophy. It also has less elastin, a type of protein present in the skin that allows it to stretch. One protein essential to normal skin structure, collagen, is actually changed in shape as a result of smoking.[10,11]

Increased Wrinkling

Several studies have verified that smoking increases the amount of wrinkling,[3,9,12] which increases with pack-years of smoking.[9] The increased risk for facial wrinkling among white smokers varies from study to study, but it is at least two to three times that of white nonsmokers.[3] The effect of smoking on wrinkling generally doesn't become apparent until middle age and may be more obvious in women than in men.[3]

In addition to having leathery-looking skin overall, smokers have very characteristic wrinkles. Most noticeable are tiny wrinkles that spread from the upper and lower lips. These are especially prominent in women who wear lipstick, as the lipstick tends to bleed into the wrinkles. "Crow's feet," the little lines around the eyes, are also accentuated in smokers.

Smokers' faces also show deep lines and numerous shallow lines on the cheeks and lower jaw. Many smokers develop hollow cheeks through the repeated muscular motion of inhaling cigarette smoke; these hollowed cheeks can cause smokers to look gaunt.[1,13]

Higher Risk of Psoriasis

Smokers have a significantly higher risk of developing psoriasis, a chronic skin condition characterized by reddish and silvery eruptions that can occur over the entire body. While psoriasis doesn't necessarily decrease a person's life span, the condition can be socially debilitating. As with wrinkling, the magnitude of the risk varies from study to study; but smokers have at least a two- to threefold increased risk over nonsmokers.[14,15]

Alcohol is also known to cause earlier onset and more severe psoriasis, and in most studies the possible contribution of alcohol to an increased risk of psoriasis has not been separated from the possible contribution of smoking. In studies in which the role of alcohol has been taken into account, however, researchers have found an increased risk of psoriasis associated with smoking in the absence of alcohol.[15]

Some, but not all, studies have found a dose-response association of smoking and psoriasis; in other words, the risk of psoriasis increases with increasing pack-years of smoking.[16] One expert estimates that smoking may precipitate as many as one quarter of all psoriasis cases and may possibly contribute to as many as half the cases of palmoplantar pustulosis,[15] a skin disease involving the hands and feet that some experts view as a form of psoriasis.

While it is not known exactly how smoking causes more psoriasis, some experts hypothesize that smoking brings about changes in one type of white blood cell, the polymorphonuclear leukocytes. Another hypothesis is that smoking may cause the body to release abnormally high levels of certain chemicals that, in excess quantities, lead to the damage characteristic of psoriasis.[17]

A quite unexpected complication—catching on fire—has befallen at least one patient with psoriasis who smoked. A classic treatment for psoriasis is the application of a substance high in a tar compound. One such compound, containing from 5 to 15 percent alcohol, is potentially flammable. Shortly after being treated with such a flammable compound, the patient in question lit a cigarette and burst into flame.[18]

Smoking and Skin Cancer
Smoking is not a cause of melanoma, a cancer of pigment-producing cells; but melanoma patients who smoke are more likely to die of their disease.[2] Four studies have found statistically significant associations between smoking and squamous cell carcinoma,[2] a skin cancer characterized by red, scaly, outlined patches.

Smoking and Acne
In one study there were fewer smokers than expected among a group of patients with severe acne.[19] Although the authors of the study postulated that smoking may protect against acne through an anti-inflammatory effect, it is unknown whether their finding could be applicable to less severe acne cases[2] or whether it could be replicated at all in well-designed studies.

References

1   Burke KE. Facial wrinkles: prevention and nonsurgical correction. *Postgrad Med* 1990;88:207–228.

2   Smith JB, Fenske NA. Cutaneous manifestations and consequences of smoking. *J Am Acad Dermatol* 1996; 34:717–732.

3   Ernster VL, Grady D, Riike R, et al. Facial wrinkling in men and women, by smoking status. *Am J Public Health* 1995;85:78–82.

4   Reus WF, Robson MC, Zachary L, Heggers JP. Acute effects of tobacco smoking on blood flow in the cutaneous micro-circulation. *Br J Plast Surg* 1984;37:213–215.

5   Waeber B, Schaller MD, Nussberger J, Bussien JP, et al. Skin blood flow reduced induced by cigarette smoking: role of vasopressin. *Am J Physiol* 1984;247:H895–901.

6   Craig S, Rees TD. The effects of smoking on experimental skin flaps in hamsters. *Plast Reconstr Surg 1985*;75:842–846.

7   Richardson D. Effects of tobacco smoke inhalation on capillary blood flow in human skin. *Arch Environ Health* 1987;42:19–25.

8   Joffe I. Cigarette smoking and facial wrinkling. *Ann Intern Med* 1991;115:659. (letter)

9   Kadunce DP, Burr R, Gress R, et al. Cigarette smoking: risk factor for premature facial wrinkling. *Ann Intern Med* 1991;114:840–844.

10 Lever WF, Schaumburg-Lever G. Histology of the skin. In: *Histopathology of Skin.* 6th ed. Philadelphia: Lippincott;1983:30–35.

11 Chen VL, Fleischmajer R, Schwartz E, et al. Immunochemistry of elastototic material in sun-damaged skin. *J Invest Dermatol* 1986;87:334–337.

12 Grady D, Ernster V. Does cigarette smoking make you ugly and old? *Amer J Epidemiol* 1992;135:839–842.

13 Davis BE, Koh HK. *Arch Dermatol* 1992;128:1106–1107.

14 Krueger GG, Duvic M. Epidemiology of Psoriasis: Clinical Issues. *J Invest Dermatol* 1994;102:14S–18S.

15 Williams HC. Smoking and psoriasis. *Br Med J* 1994;308:428–429.

16 Poikolainen K, Reunala T, Karvonen J. *Br J Dermatol* 1994;130:473–477.

17 Naldi L, Parazzini F, Brevi A. Family history, smoking habits, alcohol consumption and risk of psoriasis. *Br J Dermatol* 1992;127:212–217.

18 Fader DJ, Metzman MS. Hazards of smoking during therapy for psoriasis. *N Engl J Med* 1994;330:1541. (letter)

19 Mills CM, Peters TJ, Finlay AY. Does smoking influence acne? *Clin Experimental Dermatol* 1993;18:100–101.

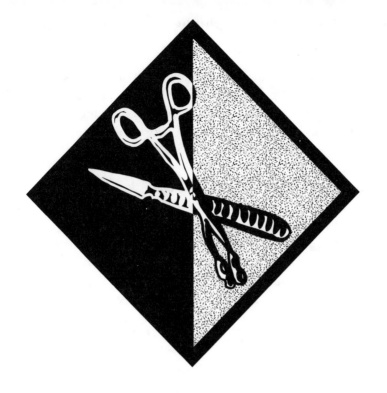

Chapter 6

SMOKING

AND SURGICAL

RISK

reviewed by
Caryl Guth, M.D.
Anesthesiologist, Mills-Peninsula Hospital
San Mateo, California
and Paul Silverstein, M.D.
Plastic Surgeon, Oklahoma City,
Oklahoma

Smoking significantly increases a person's chances of suffering complications when undergoing surgery. The risks are multiple: Smokers who require anesthesia are much more likely to suffer anesthesia-associated complications, and their surgical wounds don't heal well. Some surgeries aren't even an option for smokers.

Risk of Anesthesia Complications and Smoking

As early as 1944, experts reported that patients who smoked more than 10 cigarettes per day had a sixfold increase in postoperative respiratory complications.[1] Since that time, numerous studies have confirmed that smoking is indeed a significant risk factor for complications both during and after surgery,[2,3,4,5] and that the risk increases with pack-years of smoking.[6] The complications can be divided into three main categories:

1. an increased need for more anesthesia for a given surgical procedure;

2. an increased chance of developing a respiratory infection and other respiratory complications following surgery;

3. a lengthened stay in the recovery room and an increased need for supplemental oxygen therapy.

Smokers require more anesthesia for surgery

Among its other functions, one of the roles of anesthesia is to minimize wheezing and coughing spasms during and after surgery.[7] Because their lungs are chronically irritated,[8,9] smokers require more anesthesia for any given procedure to minimize such problems. This places them at risk of anesthesia-associated complications.

Smokers have an increased chance of respiratory infection after surgery

As noted in Chapter 1, smoking changes the mucus normally produced by the lungs and also destroys some of the cilia, the tiny hairs that beat rapidly back and forth to help clear secretions from the lungs. After a person undergoes any type of anesthesia, the ability to clear secretions is especially important. Even nonsmokers are at risk of developing pneumonia due to postoperative pain, which causes shallower breathing and ineffective coughing; and these, in turn, cause a decreased ability to clear secretions. The inability to clear secretions is magnified in smokers[6] and is associated with their much greater risk of developing respiratory infections such as pneumonia and bronchitis.[10] Smokers also have a greater chance of suffering a collapsed lung after undergoing anesthesia and surgery.[10]

Smokers have an increased length of stay in the recovery room and an increased need for supplemental oxygen after surgery
After undergoing surgery, all patients must stay in the recovery room until doctors deem their condition stable enough to allow them to return to a regular hospital room. Smokers require a significantly longer time in the recovery room to stabilize than do nonsmokers.[11] Light smokers seem to have a risk that is fairly equal to that of heavy smokers; even half-a-pack-a-day smokers suffer this complication.[12]

One of the risks following anesthesia and surgery is oxygen desaturation, an inability of the blood to carry an adequate level of oxygen. Because of this risk, oxygen is administered to patients in the recovery room after surgery.[13,14] Smoking plays a role in robbing arteries of oxygen after general anesthesia,[13] so smokers need supplemental oxygen for a longer time after surgery. Some experts even recommend that smokers continue to receive supplemental oxygen after leaving the recovery room.[13]

Does it Help to Stop Smoking Before Surgery?

Unfortunately, most people don't know they are going to have surgery until they actually need it. Most smokers don't have time to abstain from smoking for any substantial period before undergoing anesthesia. Of the 54 million smokers in the United States, about four million will undergo surgery in a given year, and most of them won't have the luxury of planning for it.[7]

Many surgeons refuse to do spinal disc surgery or any graft surgery on smokers. In the best of all worlds, a smoker who found out that he or she needed surgery would have six months to abstain from smoking. Research has indicated that patients who stopped smoking for more than six months before undergoing anesthesia had postoperative lung complications similar to those in individuals who had never smoked. In comparison, patients who stopped smoking for two months or less had a lung complication rate almost four times that of patients who had stopped for more than two months.[6]

While only long-term abstinence before surgery eliminates most complications, abstaining for even 12 or 24 hours before surgery helps eliminate or reduce carbon monoxide and nicotine from the body, thereby decreasing at least some degree of risk.[15]

Delayed Wound Healing in Smokers

The fact that smoking delays wound healing was first reported in 1977.[16] While that first report described the complication in a smoker undergoing hand surgery, multiple reports since that time have confirmed delayed wound healing in mouth surgeries[17,18]; transfer of muscle from one area of the body to another (muscle transposition)[19]; breast reconstruction[20]; face lift[21,22,23]; amputation[24]; skin graft[25,26]; spinal fusion[27]; and abdominal surgery.[28] In fact, smokers have slower healing wounds overall, whether those wounds are from surgery, injury or disease.[29]

Why Smoking Delays Wound Healing
There are at least six mechanisms by which smoking delays wound healing:

- *Smoking decreases blood flow.* As discussed in chapters 3 and 4, nicotine causes blood vessels to constrict through the same mechanism that cause the heart to beat faster and blood pressure to rise—the excessive release of body chemicals called catecholamines. That constriction reduces blood flow, thereby reducing delivery of oxygen and nutrients necessary for tissue growth, repair and maintenance.[29]

- *Smoking limits oxygen transport to a wound.* The carbon monoxide in smoke decreases the level of oxygen in the bloodstream and so decreases the amount of oxygen reaching tissues. This decrease in the level of oxygen in the blood is in addition to the reduction in blood flow described above.[29]

- *Smoking causes the release of hormones that undermine wound healing.* The smoking-induced release of catecholamines stimulates the formation of hormones called chalones. Chalones impair wound healing by slowing the rate of epithelialization, or the formation of new skin cells.[29]

- *Smoking inhibits enzyme function.* Another ingredient in cigarette smoke, hydrogen cyanide, inhibits body chemicals from working normally to transport oxygen from cell to cell, an action necessary in wound healing.[29]

- *Smoking impairs the blood-cell formation that helps healing.* In particular, nicotine reduces the formation of red blood cells, fibroblasts and macrophages. The latter two substances are important to wound healing because they transport healing substances to the wound area and are essential in scar-tissue formation.[29]

- *Smoking increases the chance that too many tiny clots will form at the wound site.* Because nicotine causes platelets (a type of blood cell necessary for normal blood clotting) to become more "sticky," smoking increases the chance that an abnormal number of clots will form at the wound site. This abnormal clotting can reduce normal blood flow to the area and thus impair healing.[29]

Smoking and Plastic Surgery

While delayed wound healing is of concern to anyone, smokers have a particularly difficult time undergoing plastic or reconstructive surgery. For this sort of surgery to be successful, flaps of skin generally must be transferred from one area of the body to another. To survive, these skin flaps depend on an adequate blood supply and enough oxygen. But because blood flow is so reduced in smokers, the skin flaps have a significantly reduced chance of survival.[29] In one study smokers undergoing plastic surgery had a 12.5 times greater risk of unsuccessful outcome of their surgery.[26] In some cases smokers may not be candidates at all for plastic or reconstructive surgery; in other cases a modified procedure may be necessary.[23,22] Smokers also need a second surgical procedure to achieve final wound healing much more often than do nonsmokers.[26]

Smoking and Hand Surgery
Smoking poses a particular problem for hand surgeries. As with other surgeries, this is because of an accumulation of smoking-induced effects on blood flow and other factors necessary for healing. Reduced blood flow is of particular concern in the hands, largely because there are so many tiny blood vessels in the hands. Smoking a single cigarette can reduce blood flow to the fingers by more than 40 percent for up to an hour.[30]

Smoking and Back Surgery
Smokers who need back surgery to fuse, or join, two vertebrae are three to four times more likely to have an unsuccessful procedure.[27] For such surgery to be successful, the bones must generate new bone cells to help fuse the vertebrae. While a nonsmoker can grow one centimeter of bone in two months, it takes ex-smokers an average of 2.5 months to grow that much new bone.[27] In active smokers, it takes an average of three months for one centimeter of bone to grow. At least one orthopedic surgeon who does such procedures will not perform them electively (that is, in a non-emergency situation) on smokers.[27]

Other Surgical Risks in Smokers
A recent study reported that smoking is one of four risk factors—the others are hypertension, previous neurological symptoms and abnormal heart rhythms—responsible for an increased risk of stroke after surgical procedures. (The researchers in this particular study looked only at people who had had surgeries not inherently associated with a high stroke risk, such as surgery to clear blocked carotid arteries.)[31]

References

1   Morton HJV. Tobacco smoking and pulmonary complications after operation. *Lancet* 1944;i:368–370. As cited in Jones RM. Smoking before surgery: the case for stopping. *Br Med J* 1985;290:1763–1764.

2   Holtz B, Bake B, Sixt R. Prediction of postoperative hypoxemia in smokers and non-smokers. *Acta Anæsth Scand* 1979;23:411–418.

3   Garibaldi RA, Britt MR, Coleman ML, et al. Risk factors for postoperative pneumonia. *Am J Med* 1981;70:677–680.

4   Mitchell C, Garrahy P, Peake P. Postoperative respiratory morbidity: identification and risk factors. *Aust NZ J Surg* 1982;52:203–209.

5   Warner MA, Divertie MB, Tinker JH. Preoperative cessation of smoking and pulmonary complications in coronary artery bypass patients. *Anesthesiology* 1984;60:380–383.

6   Warner MA, Offord MS, Warner ME, et al. Role of preoperative cessation of smoking and other factors in postoperative pulmonary complications: a blinded prospective study of coronary artery bypass patients. *Mayo Clin Proc* 1989;64:609–616.

7   Based on *Smoking Hazards and Anesthesia*. American Society of Anesthesiologists; 1989 (speech). A copy of the full text can be obtained from ASA, 520 North Northwest Highway, Park Ridge, IL 60068.

8   Lee LY, Gerhardstein DC, Wang AL, Burki NK. Nicotine is responsible for airway irritation evoked by cigarette smoke inhalation in men. *J Appl Physiol* 1993;75:1955–1961.

9   Erskine RJ, Murphy PJ, Langton JA. Sensitivity of upper airway reflexes in cigarette smokers: effect of abstinence. *Br J Anæsth* 1994;73:298–302.

10 Pearce AC, Jones RM. Smoking and anesthesia: preoperative abstinence and perioperative morbidity. *Anesthesiology* 1984;61:576–584.

11 Handlin DS, Baker T, Woolwich J. Effect of smoking on duration in recovery room. *Anesthesiology* 1990;73:A1052. Abstract.

12 Handlin DS, Baker T. The effect of heavy and light smoking on patient duration in the post anesthesia care unit. *Anesth Analg* 1991;72:S1–S336.

13 Tait AR, Kyff JV, Crider R, et al. Changes in arterial oxygen saturation in cigarette smokers following general anæsthesia. *Can J Anæsth* 1990;37:423–428.

14 Moller JT, Wittrup M, Johansen SH. Hypoxemia in the postanesthesia care unit: an observer study. *Anesthesiology* 1990;73:890–895.

15 Jones RM. Smoking before surgery: the case for stopping. *Br Med J* 1985;290:1763–1764.

16 Silverstein P. Smoking and wound healing. *Am J Med* 1992;93:1A–22S.

17 Preber H, Bergstrom J. Effect of cigarette smoking on periodontal healing following surgical therapy. *J Clin Periodontol* 1990;17:324–328.

18 Jones JK. Triplett RG. The relationship of cigarette smoking to impaired intraoral wound healing. *J Oral Maxillofac Surg* 1992;50:237–239.

19 Lovich SF, Arnold PG. The effect of smoking on muscle transposition. *Plast Reconst Surg* 1994;93:825.

20 Kroll SS. Necrosis of abdominoplasty and other secondary flaps after TRAM flap breast reconstruction. *Plast Reconst Surg* 1994;94:637–643.

21 Riefkohl R, Wolfe JA, Cox EB, McCarty KS. Association between cutaneous occlusive vascular disease, cigarette smoking and skin slough after rhytidectomy. *Plast Reconst Surg* 1986;77:592–594.

22 Webster RC, Kazda G, Hamdan US, et al. Cigarette smoking and face lift: conservative versus wide undermining. *Plast Reconst Surg* 1986;77:596–602.

23 Kaye BL. Discussion. *Plast Reconst Surg* 1986;77:603–604.

24 Lind J, Kramhoft M, Bodtker S. The influence of smoking on complications after primary amputations of the lower extremity. *Clin Orthop* 1991;267:211–217.

25 Goldminz D, Bennett RG. Cigarette smoking and flap and full-thickness graft necrosis. *Arch Dermatol* 1991;127:1012–1015.

26 Reus WF, Colen LB, Straker DJ. Tobacco smoking and complications in elective microsurgery. *Plast Reconst Surg* 1992;89:490–494.

27 Whitesides TE, Hanley EN, Fellrath FT. Smoking abstinence: is it necessary before spinal fusion. *Spine* 1994;19:2012–2014.

28 Siana JE, Rex S, Gottrup F. The effect of cigarette smoking on wound healing. *Scand J Plast Reconst Surg* 1989;23:207–209.

29 Silverstein P. Smoking and wound healing. *Am J Med* 1992;93 (suppl 1A):1A–22S.

30 Sarin CL, Austin JC, Nickel WO. Effects of smoking on digital blood flow velocity. *JAMA* 1974;229:1327–1328.

31 Parikh S, Cohen JR. Perioperative stroke after general surgical procedures. *NY State J Med* 1993;93:162–165.

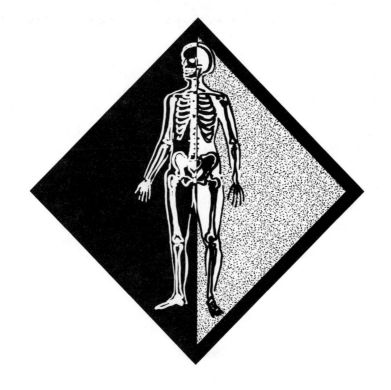

Chapter 7

SMOKING
AND ORTHOPEDIC
PROBLEMS

reviewed by
Russell Cecil, M.D.
Orthopedic Surgeon
Amsterdam,
New York

Although the bones and supporting soft tissues would seem far removed from any effects smoking might have on the body, they, too, are adversely affected. Smokers suffer more fractures because they have higher rates of osteoporosis (decreased bone density). Their fractures take longer to heal. Also, smokers are more likely to suffer back pain and musculoskeletal injuries. The association between smoking and back pain is so strong, in fact, that experts believe the prevention of back pain to be a beneficial side effect of antismoking campaigns.[1]

In this chapter we will review the effects smoking has on orthopedic problems. For information on osteoporosis and arthritic conditions, please refer to Chapter 8, on smoking and rheumatological conditions.

About Bones
The human skeleton is a constantly changing, living tissue. From the day we are born to the day we die, our bones undergo a process called remodeling, a breaking down of old bone and the replacement of it with strong, new bone. A good blood supply is critical to this process. To be healthy, bones, like any other living tissue, need the oxygen and nutrients that blood supplies. But just as smoking reduces blood flow to the heart and other critical organs, it also reduces blood flow to the bones. The consequences to the musculoskeletal system of decreased blood flow are many, as are the direct effects to that system of the chemicals in smoke.

Orthopedic Problems from Smoking: Back and Neck Trouble
There is a substantial literature reporting an association between smoking and back pain.[2] Specifically, smoking contributes to the process by which discs in the spine are weakened. These discs are pads of tissue that serve as cushions between the vertebrae, the bones that form the spine. The prevalence of back pain increases both with the number of pack-years of smoking and with heavier smoking. In other words, smokers with severe back pain generally have smoked longer and more heavily than those with moderate or no back pain.[1]

While all smokers suffer more back problems, industrial workers who smoke are even more likely to suffer low-back injuries.[3] One in two smokers experiences back pain as a result of a work-related injury, as compared with one in five nonsmokers.[4] In addition, people who smoke more than one pack per day are more handicapped by their back pain than are those who smoke less or not at all.[4]

Not only is smoking associated with more back pain, but it may also increase the likelihood that a weakened disc will rupture, a condition known as herniated disc. This effect has not been reported consistently across studies, however. Two studies reported nearly a twofold increased risk for herniated disc among smokers,[5,6] but a third study failed to find an association.[7]

Scientists have proposed more than one mechanism by which smoking might cause spinal-disc damage. First, smoking reduces blood flow to the discs, which restricts the amount of nutrients and oxygen they receive. The carbon monoxide and nicotine in cigarette smoke also have direct, adverse effects on the discs. Because the discs are compromised by these mechanisms, they are less healthy and more susceptible to injury.[2,3]

Another mechanism that may possibly cause back pain in smokers is coughing. Because coughing increases pressure in the abdominal area and also increases the pressure inside the discs, a smoker's repetitive coughing may damage discs and so cause back trouble.[1]

Surgery to treat back problems is less successful in smokers. When a patient is diagnosed with certain kinds of back trouble, he or she may need a type of surgery in which two of the vertebrae are fused, or joined together. The vertebrae in a smoker's spine are less likely to fuse successfully; those that do fuse take longer to do so. There is also evidence that whatever bone is formed in the fusion may have inferior biomechanical properties in smokers.

Experts believe that the nicotine in tobacco smoke is responsible for delayed and unsuccessful spinal fusion. The evidence for smoking-induced failure of spinal fusion is so strong that many surgeons insist that smokers quit before the procedure; some won't perform surgery unless the patient quits. The experts even call into question the use of nicotine patches to assuage withdrawal symptoms.[8] In animal models, nicotine alone causes resorption of bone at fusion sites.

Increased Risk of Musculoskeletal Injury
The bones forming the skeleton are supported by soft tissues called muscles, tendons and ligaments; together, the bones and supporting tissues are called the musculoskeletal system. Smokers suffer more injuries to the soft

tissues of the musculoskeletal system for the same reasons that they suffer more injured discs in their spinal columns: Nicotine-induced vasoconstriction (constriction of the blood vessels) reduces blood flow and limits the amounts of oxygen and nutrients reaching the soft tissues. As a result, they are less healthy and more susceptible to injury.[3,9]

Broken Bones
Smokers suffer more fractures than do nonsmokers, and their fractures take longer to heal. The difference in healing rates between smokers and nonsmokers is dramatic: A nonsmoker's broken leg heals an average of 80 percent faster than a smoker's broken leg. Expressed as the number of days necessary for healing, an average smoker's bones take 276 days to heal; a nonsmoker's, 146 days.[10]

While the research isn't conclusive, experts theorize that reduced blood flow interferes with bone healing in smokers.[10] This theory is supported by research in which bone grafts implanted into rabbits who were subsequently exposed to nicotine did not "take," or become incorporated into the rabbits' own bone, as well as did grafts implanted into rabbits not exposed to nicotine.[11] Other experts theorize that nicotine has a direct detrimental effect on osteoclasts, the cells that facilitate the incorporation of new bony tissue to heal a fracture. It appears that nicotine causes osteoblasts to make DNA, the blueprint for new cells, too quickly. In turn, the new osteoblasts produced aren't normal and so cannot facilitate the incorporation of new bony tissue to help repair the fracture.[11]

Less Successful Orthopedic Surgeries
In addition to interfering with back surgery, smoking thwarts the success of other orthopedic surgeries. To repair some fractures or reconstruct bone from which tumors have been removed, orthopedic surgeons sometimes must graft donor bone to the injured or diseased area. In smokers, however, these bone grafts are less likely to become incorporated into the patient's own bone. Again, nicotine-induced vasoconstriction leading to reduced blood supply is thought to be responsible.[12]

References

1   Boshuizen HC, Verbeek JHAM, Broersen JPJ, Weel ANH. Do smokers get more back pain? *Spine* 1993;18:35–40.

2   Ernst E. Smoking, a cause of back trouble? *Br J Rheumatol* 1993;32:239–242.

3   Tsai SP, Gilstrap EL, Cowles SR, Waddell LC, Ross CE. Personal and job characteristics of musculoskeletal injuries in an industrial population. *J Occupational Med* 1992;34: 606–612.

4   Hanley EH, Kane SM, Bohren BF, et al. Healthy lifestyle and low back pain. Presented at the 1995 Annual AAOS Meeting, Orlando, FL. Paper #304.

5   Heliovaara M, Knekt P, Aromaa A. Incidence and risk factors of herniated lumbar intervertebral disc or sciatica leading to hospitalization. *J Chron Dis* 1987;40:251–258.

6   Kelsey JL, Githens PB, O'Conner T, et al. Acute prolapsed lumbar intervertebral disc. An epidemiological study with special reference to driving automobiles and cigarette smoking. *Spine* 1984;9:608–613.

7   Kelsey JL. An epidemiological study of acute herniated lumbar intervertebral discs. *Rheumatol Rehabil* 1975;14:144–159.

8   Silcox DH, Daftari T, Boden SD, Schimandle JH, Hutton WC, Whitesides TE. The effect of nicotine on spinal fusion. *Spine* section, Dept. of Orthopedic Surgery, Emory University School of Medicine.   Presented at the 1995 Annual AAOS Meeting, Orlando, FL. Paper #269.

9   Ekberg K, Bjorkqvist B, Malm P, Bjerre-Kiely B, Karlsson M, Axelson O. Case-control study of risk factors for disease in the neck and shoulder area. *Occupational and Environmental Med* 1994;54:262–266.

10   Schmitz MA, Finnegan M, Champine J, Jones A. The effect of smoking on the clinical healing of tibial shaft fractures. 1995 study released by the University of Texas at Dallas, Parkland Memorial Hospital, Departments of Orthopedics and Radiology.

11   Schmitz MA, Finnegan M, Champine J, Jones A. The effect of smoking on the clinical healing of tibial shaft fractures. Presented at the 1995 Annual AAOS Meeting, Orlando, FL. Paper #498.

12   Riebel GD, Boden SD, Whitesides TE, Hutton WC. The effect of nicotine on incorporation of cancellous bone graft in an animal model. Published through Department of Orthopedic Surgery, Emory University School of Medicine, Atlanta, GA.

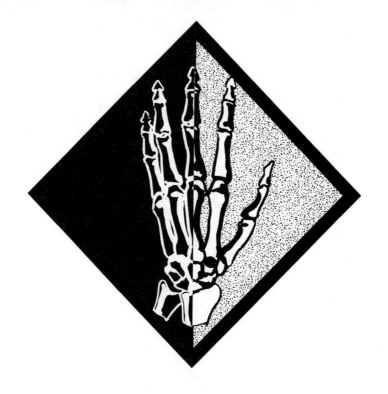

Chapter 8

SMOKING

AND RHEUMATOLOGIC

CONDITIONS

reviewed by
Robert G. Lahita, M.D., Ph.D.
Associate Professor, Columbia University
Chief of Rheumatology, St. Luke's-Roosevelt
Medical Center, New York,
New York

Rheumatology is the study of conditions that affect the joints, including the many forms of arthritis and osteoporosis. The most noticeable impact of smoking in this realm is an increased risk for osteoporosis, a reduction in bone mass. There is also some evidence that smoking increases the smoker's risk for developing rheumatoid arthritis. For reasons explained below, smoking may actually protect against osteoarthritis of the large joints.

In this chapter we review the impact of smoking on rheumatologic conditions. For information on orthopedic problems—including descriptions of how smoking interferes with the healing of fractures, increases the risk for back trouble and magnifies the risk for suffering musculoskeletal injury—please refer to Chapter 7.

Increased Risk of Osteoporosis

Osteoporosis forever changes its victims' lifestyles and physical abilities. It causes bones to become weak, porous and subject to fracture. Women are the primary victims of osteoporosis (as many as half of American women over age 45 have it), but elderly men are also frequently affected. Osteoporosis can even lead to death: As many as 20 percent of people who suffer a hip fracture—one consequence of osteoporosis—die within a year of the fracture from associated complications, such as pneumonia or a blood clot. Both pneumonia and blood clots can develop as a result of the immobility associated with a fractured hip.

There are many risk factors for developing osteoporosis. They include a diet low in calcium and vitamin D, a lack of exercise, thinness—and cigarette smoking. Smoking contributes to osteoporosis by depleting bones of the minerals, especially calcium, that help keep them strong and dense.[1] The bone mineral content of male smokers averages about 10 to 20 percent less than that of nonsmokers; the bone mineral content of women smokers averages 15 to 30 percent less than that of nonsmokers.[2]

One investigator found X-ray evidence that certain bones in the hands of female smokers are 50 percent less dense than the same bones in similar-aged nonsmoking women.[2] In another study women who smoked one pack of cigarettes per day throughout their adult life had a 5 to 10 percent deficit in bone mass by the time they reached menopause. This is enough of a deficit to increase fracture risk substantially.[3]

One study found that for every 10 pack-years of smoking, bone density in smokers, as compared with nonsmokers, was 2.0 percent lower at the lumbar spine, 0.9 percent lower at the femoral neck (the top of the thigh bone) and 1.4 percent lower at the femoral shaft (the other end of the thigh bone).[3] The smoking-osteoporosis association is dose-dependent in both men and women, with the condition worsening as smoking increases.[4]

Unfortunately, it doesn't take a lifetime of smoking to increase the risk for brittle bones. A recent, disturbing study reported that teenage girls who smoke have a lower bone mineral density than similar-aged girls who don't smoke.[5] This means that smoking teenagers are less likely to achieve the highest peak bone mass possible (bones stop growing in length relatively early in life, but they increase in density through the third decade). Not achieving the highest possible peak bone mass is yet another risk factor for osteoporosis.

Osteoporosis is commonly considered a woman's disease (and women *do* suffer more osteoporosis than men); but, as previously mentioned, men also suffer brittle bones. Approximately one fourth of hip fractures occur in men; one in six white men who reach their 80s will suffer a hip fracture.[6] Smoking is a moderate risk factor for osteoporosis in men, with male smokers having a risk nearly two and a half times that of their nonsmoking counterparts.[6,7] This is approximately the same increase in risk experienced by women who smoke as compared with their nonsmoking peers.[1]

One of the ways smoking robs bones of strength-lending minerals is by decreasing the amount of estrogen in the body. This mechanism applies to men as well as women. Men's estrogen levels are much lower than women's, but the estrogen in men's bodies is still important for retaining calcium in bones. Among its many other functions, estrogen helps bones "hold on" to calcium and other minerals that lend strength to bones.

At menopause a woman's body produces much less estrogen, so every postmenopausal woman is at elevated risk for osteoporosis. During and after menopause many women take hormone replacement therapy, which includes estrogen, both to relieve hot flashes and other symptoms of menopause and to protect against heart disease and osteoporosis. Replacing estrogen after menopause decreases a woman's chances of developing osteoporosis, but the replacement estrogen cannot do its job properly in postmenopausal women who smoke. Not only does estrogen not protect postmenopausal smokers against osteoporosis and its resultant fractures, but the estrogen may actually increase postmenopausal smokers' risk of developing a blood clot *because they smoke.*[8]

Smoking also makes bones more brittle by interfering with the metabolism of vitamin D.[2] Without vitamin D the body cannot absorb adequate calcium, and calcium is the most important mineral dictating bone strength. Calcium is absorbed in the small intestine into cells called enterocytes. Vitamin D plays two roles in this absorptive process: It regulates the process and it is a necessary ingredient in the protein that transports the calcium across the membrane of the enterocytes.

Smoking also increases osteoporosis risk indirectly because smokers tend to exercise less than nonsmokers.[9] Exercise helps the bones hang on to calcium and other minerals; thus, it is critical to helping bones stay strong. But extensive studies have verified that smokers are less physically active than nonsmokers.[10,11]

Smokers, as a group, are also thinner than nonsmokers; and leanness is another risk factor for osteoporosis.[12] The risk of hip fracture in thin women who smoke jumps to four times that of their nonsmoking, less thin counterparts.[1]

As noted above, people with osteoporosis have a greater risk of suffering fractures; they also suffer more disability. In a study of 9,704 older women, lifetime cigarette consumption was associated with impaired functioning and impaired mobility. Current smokers in the study were more likely to report impaired function, and an increasing number of pack-years was associated with a greater risk of disability.[13]

Smoking and Rheumatoid Arthritis: A Tenuous Association

Rheumatoid arthritis is a chronic condition in which the joints, especially those of the hands and feet, become painful and deformed. In addition, the body's vital organs—including the lungs—can become involved. There is a substantial literature exploring the association between smoking and rheumatoid arthritis; most investigators report a tenuous association at best.

In one study of over 17,000 women, those who smoked were nearly 2 1/2 times as likely as nonsmokers to have rheumatoid arthritis.[14] Other studies have found less dramatic increased risks for developing rheumatoid arthritis.[15,16] At least three studies have found an increased risk for men but not for women.[17,18,19] Still other studies have failed to find any association, however, and at least one study found that smoking actually protects against developing rheumatoid arthritis.[20]

If an association exists between smoking and rheumatoid arthritis, there are at least two possible mechanisms. One investigator found that smokers are more likely to have high blood levels of antinuclear antibodies (ANA), an immunologic abnormality. While high ANA levels are associated with rheumatoid arthritis and other rheumatologic conditions,[17] the relationship between positive ANA and smoking remains unclear. For unknown reasons, in people with rheumatoid arthritis and some other rheumatologic conditions, the immune system turns the body against itself, reacting to its own tissues as if they were foreign substances and making antibodies that attack them.

Another possible mechanism that could explain a smoking and rheumatoid arthritis association involves the roles played by carbon monoxide, cyanide, tars and other toxins in cigarette smoke in inducing the immunologic abnormalities that trigger rheumatoid arthritis.[21]

One finding that is not tenuous is the fact that smoking *worsens* certain manifestations of rheumatoid arthritis. In patients whose rheumatoid arthritis causes lung problems, including impaired lung function, smoking is likely to increase the severity of those problems.[17]

Protection Against Osteoarthritis

Osteoarthritis is the most common joint disease and the leading cause of disability in the elderly; it is commonly thought of as the arthritis of aging.

There is some evidence that smoking protects against osteoarthritis of the large joints, in particular the knee, with the heaviest smokers having the lowest risk.[22,23] While results aren't consistent, some studies indicate that heavy smokers have only half the risk of nonsmokers of developing osteoarthritis of the knee.[24] Although people who weigh more are more apt to develop osteoarthritis of the knee, and smokers are generally thinner, differences in body weight failed to account for this apparent protective effect.

One proposed mechanism is that because the bones of smokers are less dense, they are more pliable. This pliability spares the cartilage at the joints from becoming damaged and could therefore minimize changes that lead to osteoarthritis. Alternatively, smoking may influence immune system components that enhance arthritic changes, such as immunoregulatory T cells and macrophages (see Chapter 19, Smoking and the Immune System, for more detail on these immune-system components).[24]

Yet another mechanism suggests that smoking may exert some direct, positive effect on chondrocytes, the cells that make up cartilage, thereby reducing the changes that lead to osteoarthritis.[23]

Increased Risk for Heberden's Nodules

Although smoking may be protective against osteoarthritis, smokers with the disease are at greater risk of developing Heberden's nodules, bony bumps about the size of a pea (or smaller) that sometimes develop on the top part of the fingers in people who have osteoarthritis. In at least one study, smokers with osteoarthritis were about twice as likely to develop Heberden's nodules as were nonsmoking osteoarthritis patients.[25] These nodules can become quite swollen and painful and can cause considerable disability.

References

1   LaVecchia CL, Negri E, Levi F, Baron JA. Cigarette smoking, body mass and other risk factors for fractures of the hip in women. *International J Epidemiol* 1991;20:671–677.

2   Rundgren A, Mellstrom D. The effect of tobacco smoking on the bone mineral content of the ageing skeleton. *Mechanisms of Ageing and Development* 1984;28:273–277.

3   Hopper JL, Seeman E. The bone density of female twins discordant for tobacco use. *N Engl J Med* 1994;330:387–392.

4   Hollenbach KA, Barrett-Connor E, Edelstein SL, Holbrook T. Cigarette smoking and bone mineral density in older men and women. *Am J Public Health* 1993;83:1265–1270.

5   Turner J, Gilchrist N, Ayling E, et al. Factors affecting bone mineral density in high school girls. *N Zealand Med J* 1992;105:95–96.

6   Niewoehner CB. Osteoporosis in men: is it more common than we think? *Postgrad Med* 1993;93:59–70.

7   Slemenda CW, Christian JC, Reed T, et al. Long-term bone loss in men: effects of genetic and environmental factors. *Ann Intern Med* 1992;117:286–291.

8   Ali N, Twibell R (review article) Perimenopausal and elderly women report osteoporosis-preventive behaviors and the perceptions related to performing those behaviors. *Geriatric Nursing* 1994;15:201–205.

9   McCulloch RG, Whiting SJ, Bailey DA, Houston CS. The effect of cigarette smoking on trabecular bone density in premenopausal women aged 20–35 years. *Can J Public Health* 1991;82:434–435.

10   Blair S, Jacobs D, Powell KE. Relationships between exercise or physical activity and other health behaviors. *Public Health Rep* 1985;100:172–180.

11   Marks BL, Perkins KA, Metz KF, et al. Effects of smoking status on content of caloric intake and energy expenditure. *International Journal on Eating Disorders* 1991;10:441–449.

12   LaCroix AZ, Omenn GS. Older adults and smoking. *Health Promotion and Disease Prevention* 1992;8:69–87.

13   Ensrud KE, Nevitt MC, Yunis C, et al. Correlates of impaired function in older women. *J Am Geriatrics Soc* 1994;42:481–489.

14   Vessey MP, Villard-Mackintosh L, Yeates D. Oral contraceptives, cigarette smoking and other factors in relation to arthritis. *Contraception* 1987;35:457–464.

15 Fischer KM. Hypothesis: tobacco use is a risk factor in rheumatoid arthritis. *Med Hypotheses* 1991;34:116–117.

16 Hernandez-Avila M, Liang M, Willett WC, et al. Reproductive factors, smoking and the risk for rheumatoid arthritis. Epidemiology 1990;1:285–291.

17 Tuomi T, Heliovaara M, Palosuo T, Aho K. Smoking, lung function and rheumatoid arthritis. *Annals of the Rheumatic Diseases* 1990;49:753–756.

18 Heliovaara M, Aho K, Aromas A, et al. Smoking and risk of rheumatoid arthritis. *J Rheumatol* 1993;20:1830–1835.

19 Mathews JD, Whittingham S, Hooper BM, Mackay JR. Association of autoantibodies with smoking, cardiovascular morbidity, and death in the Busselton population. *Lancet* 1973;2:754–758.

20 Hazes JMW, Dijkmans BAC, Vandenbroucke JP, et al. Lifestyle and the risk of rheumatoid arthritis: cigarette smoking and alcohol consumption. *Annals of the Rheumatic Diseases* 1990;49:980–982.

21 Silman AJ. Smoking and the risk of rheumatoid arthritis. *J Rheumatol* 1993;20:11–12.

22 Anderson JJ, Felson DT. Factors associated with osteoarthritis of the knee in the first national health and nutrition examination survey. Evidence for an association with overweight, race and physical demands of the work. *Am J Epidemiol* 1988;128:179–189.

23 Felson DT, Anderson JJ, Naimark A, et al. Does smoking protect against osteoarthritis? *Arthritis Rheum* 1989;166–172.

24 Samanta A, Jones A, Regan M, et al. Is osteoarthritis in women affected by hormonal changes or smoking? *Br J Rheumatol* 1993;32:366–370.

25 Hart DJ, Spector TD. Cigarette smoking and risk of osteoarthritis in women in the general population: the Chingford study. *Ann Rheum Dis* 1993;52:93–96.

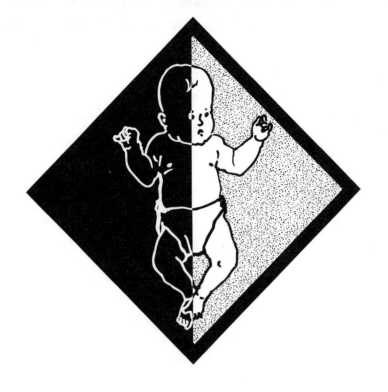

Chapter 9

ENVIRONMENTAL
TOBACCO SMOKE
AND PEDIATRIC
ILLNESSES

reviewed by
Miles M. Weinberger, M.D.
Professor of Pediatrics and Chairman,
Pediatric Allergy and Pulmonary Division,
University of Iowa Hospitals
and Clinics

The 1988 National Health Interview Survey on Child Health estimated that 42 percent of children aged five and under live in households with current smokers.[1] The Third National Health and Nutrition Examination Survey (1988 to 1991) estimated that almost 88 percent of nonusers of tobacco have detectable blood levels of cotinine, a metabolic by-product of nicotine.[2]

According to the Environmental Protection Agency (EPA), children's "passive smoking," as it is called, results in hundreds of thousands of cases of bronchitis, pneumonia, ear infections and worsened asthma. Worse yet, the Centers for Disease Control and Prevention estimates that 702 children younger than one year die each year as a result of passive smoking: they die from sudden infant death syndrome (SIDS), worsened asthma and serious respiratory infections.[3]

In this chapter we review the multiple and serious consequences of children's exposure to environmental tobacco smoke. (Please refer to Chapter 10, Smoking and Complications in Obstetrics and Gynecology, for a summary of the smoking-induced complications inflicted upon developing and newborn babies). We begin this chapter with definitions of the smoking by-products children inhale when they are around smokers.

Definitions of Tobacco Smoke

There are three types of tobacco smoke: mainstream smoke, sidestream smoke and environmental tobacco smoke. Mainstream smoke (MS) is the smoke inhaled by smokers. It is generated during puffs and passes through the butt end of the cigarette. Sidestream smoke (SS) is the smoke freshly generated by a passively burning cigarette and emitted directly into the air; it does not include exhaled particles from smokers. Approximately 80 percent of a cigarette's tobacco is burned passively.[4] Environmental tobacco smoke (ETS) is a mixture of sidestream and exhaled mainstream smokes,[5] as well as contaminants that diffuse through the cigarette paper and mouth end of the cigarette between puffs.[6] In the remainder of this chapter, we refer to the smoke inhaled by children exposed to smokers as ETS.

ETS is very similar to MS; it contains more than 3,800 chemical compounds.[7] Surprisingly, SS generally has a more highly carcinogenic mix than does MS. This is because SS usually has more contaminants than MS.[8] SS also differs from MS in that the toxic products in SS may be in a different physical form.[5] Nicotine, for example, occurs predominantly in the solid particle phase in MS but in the gas phase in ETS.[9]

Particle size varies in the different types of tobacco smoke. The size of solid particles ranges from 0.1 to 1.0 micrometers in MS but from 0.01 to 1.0 micrometers in SS. Also, as sidestream smoke becomes more dilute, the particle sizes become smaller.[6,10] Because the particles in sidestream smoke are generally smaller than the particles in MS, they reach deeper sections of the lung[4,11] (by definition, then, the particles in ETS are also smaller than mainstream particles).

Evidence that ETS Damages Health

There is overwhelming evidence that the constituents of environmental tobacco smoke damage health in those passively exposed.

Consider the following:

- Many of the constituents of mainstream cigarette smoke are present in reduced quantities in the smoke exhaled by active smokers, which is then inhaled by others.[12] Despite the fact that these levels are small, active smoking increases cancer risk even at low doses, such as five to 10 cigarettes per day. Reliable studies of active smokers show that there is no threshold below which active smoking ceases to pose an increased risk of lung cancer.[13] Many experts believe that exposure to ETS results in health risks that are similar to being a light active smoker.[14]

- Some chemicals appear in higher concentration in SS than in MS.[12] Included among the long list of chemicals generally found in higher concentrations in SS are 3-vinylpyridine, N-nitrosodimethylamine, N-nitrosodiethylamine, nicotine, 2-naphthylamine, 4-amino-biphenyl and polonium-210.[8]

- The argument that passive inhalation is less hazardous than primary smoking because smoke enters through the nose rather than being taken directly into the lungs has now been dismissed, because researchers have found that ETS particles are so small that they escape the nasal filtering system and enter the lungs directly. And, as noted above, ETS particles are smaller than mainstream particles. As a result, they generally penetrate deeper into lung tissue than does the smoke that smokers inhale.[4,11]

- Passive smoking is related primarily to those forms of lung cancer that show the highest relative risks in smokers: squamous cell and small cell carcinomas.[15,16,17,18]

Health Consequences

Children exposed to their parents' tobacco smoke suffer significant respiratory diseases. The most pronounced risk is for infants under one year of age.[19,20,21] Experts suspect that younger lung tissue is more vulnerable to insult and is subject to damage at lower concentrations of contaminants, including a relatively low concentration of ETS. The younger the child, the more serious the consequences of ETS exposure with increasing doses of exposure.[22]

Many studies have shown that maternal smoking poses a greater risk for infants' respiratory illness than does paternal smoking because mothers are more commonly at home than are fathers. This finding suggests that the duration of the exposure, rather than simply the presence of a smoker in the house, is an important factor in infant respiratory disease.[19,23]

Lower Respiratory-Tract Infections

Children exposed to passive smoke have an increased risk of lower respiratory-tract infections, including bronchitis and pneumonia.[21,24,25] Experts estimate that between 150,000 and 300,000 cases of bronchitis and pneumonia annually are attributable to ETS in children up to 18 months of age.[8] During the first year of life children of smokers are twice as likely to suffer bronchitis, pneumonia and other lower respiratory-tract illnesses as compared with children of nonsmokers.[7] In addition, children of smokers who suffer these illnesses have far more serious cases and must spend 20 percent more time in bed to recover.[26] Finally, ETS-exposed children who get pneumonia and bronchitis also have a 20 to 40 percent increased risk for hospitalization to treat their infections.[24,27,28,29]

Increased Incidence and Severity of Asthma

Parental smoking, and especially maternal smoking, is associated with an increase in the incidence and severity of asthma.[30,31,32,33,34,35,36,37] Exposure to ETS is also a risk factor for a child to develop a new case of asthma.[8] According to the American Academy of Pediatrics (AAP), exposure to the smoke of as few as 10 cigarettes per day raises a child's chance of getting asthma, even if that child has never had any symptoms before. [38]

Compared with asthmatic children from nonsmoking households, asthmatic children of smoking parents require more medications[30] and have nearly a doubled risk of having asthma that impairs their everyday functioning.[34] Asthmatic children of smokers also require more trips to the hospital to resolve their asthma attacks than do children of nonsmokers. Overall, it is estimated that anywhere from 200,000 to as many as one million asthmatic children are adversely affected by their parents' smoking.[8]

Acute and Chronic Middle-Ear Diseases

Exposure to ETS also increases the risk of chronic infections and fluid in the middle ear.[7,29,39,40] Middle-ear infections not only impose a tremendous economic burden but may cause lifelong hearing loss.[41,42] Hearing loss beginning at an early age can have serious consequences on a child's ability to speak and learn.

Many children with chronic middle-ear infections need ear tubes to drain excess fluid that accumulates in the middle ear. While some children need only one tube (or set of tubes) to resolve the problem, children of smokers need to have the tube (or tubes) replaced far more frequently than do children of nonsmokers.[43] Such tubes must be placed surgically while the child is under general anesthesia, itself a risk. In addition, repeated tube insertion can cause scarring in the middle ear, which can cause or contribute to hearing loss.

Other Respiratory-Tract Illnesses

Children exposed to ETS have more sore throats, stuffy noses, hoarseness and trouble getting over colds than do unexposed children. ETS-exposed children also undergo more adenoidectomies (removal of the adenoids) and tonsillectomies (removal of the tonsils).[44] Experts note that the need for tonsillectomy correlates with a history of more frequent upper respiratory-tract disease.[45]

Children of smokers are also 30 to 80 percent more likely than children of nonsmoking parents to have chronic cough or phlegm production. This is especially true for infants and preschool children, who are exposed for longer periods of each day than are school-aged children.[7,46,47]

Cardiovascular Effects

Passive smoking in children can lead to a variety of effects on the cardiovascular system. These effects include impaired delivery of oxygen to body tissues; a blunted heart rate response to exercise; and a chronic, mildly increased heart rate.[48]

Heavy-Metal Exposure

Passive smoking also plays an important role in exposing children to lead, a component of tobacco smoke. Parental smoking is directly related to children's blood lead levels,[49] with children of heavier smokers having higher lead levels than children of lighter smokers.

Sudden Infant Death Syndrome

Several studies, the first reported as early as 1966, provide compelling evidence that children of smoking mothers have an increased risk of sudden infant death syndrome, or SIDS. SIDS, which is also called crib death, is the most frequent cause of death in infants aged one month to one year. SIDS claims approximately 5,000 lives annually.[50,51,52,53,54,55,56,57] A 1995 report estimated that as many as 30 percent of SIDS cases might be prevented if mothers didn't smoke.[58] (For more on smoking and SIDS, see page 87.)

Gastrointestinal Diseases

Compared with children not exposed to secondhand smoke at all, children exposed to ETS after birth have a 5.3 times increased risk of developing Crohn's disease.

Crohn's disease is a chronic, inflammatory bowel condition in which patients suffer bouts of severe diarrhea and intestinal bleeding, problems that originate in either or both the small and large intestines. Many times, the disease becomes so severe that Crohn's patients must have part of their intestine removed; some people go through multiple surgeries. Passive smoking increases the risk of developing Crohn's disease, and the risk increases with the amount of passive smoke exposure.

There is also an association between passive smoke exposure during pregnancy and Crohn's disease, but it is not as strong as passive smoke exposure after birth.[59] (For more on smoking and Crohn's disease, see Chapter 18.)

Passive smoking is also a risk factor for developing another chronic bowel condition, ulcerative colitis. This condition, which affects only the large bowel, causes bouts of severe diarrhea and bleeding. Children exposed to ETS have more than a doubled risk of developing ulcerative colitis as compared with unexposed children. The risk is much greater for children exposed after birth than it is for children exposed in utero.[59]

References

1   Overpeck MD, Moss AJ. Children's exposure to environmental cigarette smoke before and after birth. Advance Data from Vital and Health Statistics of the National Center for Health Statistics #202. DHHS Pub. No. (PHS) 91–1250; 1991.

2   Pirkle JL, Flegal KM, Bernert JT, Brody DJ, Etzel RA, Maurer KR. Exposure of the US population to environmental tobacco smoke: The Third National Health and Nutrition Examination Survey, 1988 to 1991. *JAMA* 1996;275:1233–1240.

3   *MMWR* 1991;40:62–71.

4   Blot WJ, Fraumeni JF. Passive smoking and lung cancer. *JNCI* 1986;77:993–1000.

5   Smith CJ, Sears SB, Walker JC, DeLuca P, *Toxicologic Pathology* 1992;20:289–305.

6   Guerin MR, Jenkins RA, Tomkins BA. *The Chemistry of Environmental Tobacco Smoke: Composition and Measurement.* Chelsea, MI: Lewis Publishers, 1992.

7   Committee on Passive Smoking, Board of Environmental Studies and Toxicology, National Research Council. *Environmental Tobacco Smoke: Measuring Exposures and Assessing Health Effects.* Washington, DC: National Academy Press, 1986.

8   US Environmental Protection Agency. *Respiratory Health Effects of Passive Smoking: Lung Cancer and Other Disorders.* 1992.

9   Eudy LW, Thorne, FA, Heavor, DL, Green CR, Ingebrethsen BJ, 1985, as cited in *Respiratory Health Effects of Passive Smoking: Lung Cancer and Other Disorders,* US EPA, 1992.

10 US Department of Health and Human Services. *The Health Consequences of Involuntary Smoking: A Report of the Surgeon General,* 1986.

11 Heath CW. Passive smoking: environmental tobacco smoke and lung cancer. *Lancet* 1993;341:526.

12 Peto J, Doll R. Passive smoking: guest editorial. *Br J Cancer* 1986;54:381–383.

13 *The Health Consequences of Smoking: Cancer, a Report of the Surgeon General.* Washington, DC: Government Printing Office, 1982. Pub. No. DHHS (PHS) 82–50179.

14 Blot WJ, Fraumeni JF. Guest editorial: passive smoking and lung cancer. *JNCI* 1986;77:993–1000.

15 Pershagen G, Hrubec Z, Svensson C. Passive smoking and lung cancer in Swedish women. *Am J Epidemiol* 1987;125:17–24.

16 Gao YT, Blot WJ, Zheng W, et al. Lung cancer among Chinese women. *Int J Cancer* 1987;40:604–609.

17 Dalager NA, Pickle LW, Mason TJ, et al. The relation of passive smoking to lung cancer. Cancer Research 1986;46:4808–4811.

18 Doll R, Hill AB, Kreyberg L. The significance of cell type in relation to the etiology of lung cancer. *Br J Cancer* 1957;11:43–48.

19 Pedreira FA, Guandolo VL, Feroli EJ. Involuntary smoking and incidence of respiratory illness during the first year of life. *Pediatrics* 1985;75:594–595.

20 Colley JRT, Holland WW, Corkhill RT. Influence of passive smoking and parental phlegm on pneumonia and bronchitis in early childhood. *Lancet* 1974;1:1031–1034.

21 Leeder SR, et al. Influence of family factors on the incidence of lower respiratory illness during the first year of life. *Br J Prev Soc Med* 1976;30:203–212.

22 Guyatt GH, Newhouse MT. Are active and passive smoking harmful? Determining causation. *Chest* 1985;88:445–451.

23 Harlap S, Davies AM. Infant admissions to hospital and maternal smoking. *Lancet* 1974;i:529–532.

24 Fergusson DM, Horwood LJ, Shannon FT, Taylor B. Parental smoking and lower respiratory illness in the first years of life. *Journal of Epidemiology and Community Health* 1981;35:180–184.

25 Fergusson DM, Horwood LJ, Shannon FT. Parental smoking and respiratory illness in infancy. *Arch Dis Child* 1980;55:358–361.

26 Ostro BD. Estimating the risks of smoking, air pollution, and passive smoke on acute respiratory conditions. *Risk Analysis* 1989;9:189–196.

27 Chen Y, Wanxian L, Shunzhang Y. Influence of passive smoking on admissions for respiratory illness in early childhood. *Br Med J* 1986;293:303–306.

28 Harlap S, Davies AM. Infant admissions to hospital and maternal smoking. *Lancet* 1974;i:529–532.

29 *The Health Consequences of Involuntary Smoking. A Report of the Surgeon General.* US DHHS, Public Health Service, Office of the Assistant Secretary for Health, Office of Smoking and Health, Washington, DC. DHHS Pub. No. (PHS) 87-8398.

30 Weitzman M, Gortmaker S, Walker DK, Sobol A. Maternal smoking and childhood asthma. *Pediatrics* 1990;85:505–511.

31 Weiss ST, Tager IB, Speizer FE, et al. Persistent wheeze: its relation to respiratory illness, cigarette smoking and level of pulmonary function in a population sample of children. *Am Rev Resp Dis* 1980;122:697–707.

32 Ware JH, Dockery DW, Spiro A, et al. Passive smoking, gas cooking and respiratory health of children living in six cities. *Am Rev Respir Dis* 1984;129:366–374.

33 Burchfiel CM, Higgins MW, Keller JB, et al. Passive smoking in childhood: respiratory conditions and pulmonary function in Tecumseh, Michigan. *Am Rev Respir Dis* 1986;133:966–973.

34 Gortmaker SL, Walker DK, Jacobs FH et al. Parental smoking and the risk of childhood asthma. *Am J Public Health* 1982;72:574–579.

35 Evans D, Levison J, Feldman CH, et al. The impact of passive smoking on emergency room visits of urban children with asthma. *Am Rev Respir Dis* 1987;135:567–572.

36 Krzyzanowski M, Quackenboss JJ, Lebowitz MD. Chronic respiratory effects of indoor formaldehyde exposure. *Environ Res* 1990;52:117–125.

37 O'Connor GT, Weiss ST, Tager IB, et al. The effect of passive smoking on pulmonary function and non-specific bronchial responsiveness in a population based sample of children and young adults. *Am Rev Respir Dis* 1987;137:800–804.

38 American Academy of Pediatrics. *Environmental Tobacco Smoke: A Danger to Children.* 1994.

39 Etzel RA, Pattishall EN, Haley NJ, et al. Passive smoking and middle ear effusion among children in day care. *Pediatrics* 1992;90:228–232.

40 Fleming DW, Cochi SL, Hightower AW, et al. Childhood upper respiratory tract infections: to what degree is incidence affected by day-care attendance? *Pediatrics* 1987;79:55–60.

41 Maran AGD, Wilson JA. Glue ear and speech development. *Br Med J* 1986;293:713–714.

42 Black N. Surgery for glue ear—a modern epidemic? *Lancet* 1984;1:835–837.

43 Maw AR, Bawden R. Does adenoidectomy have an adjuvant effect on ventilation tube insertion and thus reduce the need for re-treatment? *Clin Otolaryngol* 1994;19:340–343.

44 Willatt DJ. Children's sore throats related to parental smoking. *Clin Otolaryngol* 1986;11:317–321.

45 Said, G, Zalokar J, Lellouch J, Patois E. Parental smoking related to adenoidectomy and tonsillectomy in children. *Journal of Epidemiology and Community Health.* 1978;32:97–101

46 Tsimoyianis GV, Jacobson MS, Feldman JG. Reduction in pulmonary function and increased frequency of cough associated with passive smoking in teenage athletes. *Pediatrics* 1987;80:32–36.

47 Bisgaard H, Kalgaard P, Nyboe J. Risk factors for wheezing during infancy: a study of 5953 infants. *Acta Pædiatr Scand* 1987;76:719–726.

48 Gidding SS, Schydlower M. Active and passive tobacco exposure: a serious pediatric health problem. *Pediatrics* 1994;94:750–751.

49 Andren P, et al. Environmental exposure to lead and arsenic among children living near a glassworks. *Sci Total Environ* 1988;77:25–34.

50 Bergman AB, Wiesner BA. Relationship of passive cigarette smoking to sudden infant death syndrome. *Pediatrics* 1976;58:665–668.

51 Hoffman HJ, Damus K, Hillman L, Krongrad E. Risk factors for SIDS. Results of the National Institute of Child Health and Human Development SIDS Cooperative Epidemiological Study. *Ann NY Acad Sci* 1988;533:13–30.

52 Haglund B, Cnattingius S. Cigarette smoking as a risk factor for sudden infant death syndrome: a population-based study. *Am J Public Health* 1990;80:29–32.

53 Lewak N, van den Berg BJ, Beckwith JB. Sudden infant death syndrome risk factors. *Clin Pediatr* (Phila) 1979;18:404–411.

54 Malloy MH, Kleinman JC, Land GH, Schramm WF. The association of maternal smoking with age and cause of infant death. *Am J Epidemiol* 1988;128:46–55.

55 Mitchell EA, Scragg R, Stewart AW, et al. Results from the first year of the New Zealand cot death study. *NA Med J* 1991;104:71–76.

56 Steele R, Landworth JT. The relationship of antenatal and postnatal factors to sudden unexpected death in infancy. *Can Med Assoc J* 1966;94:1165–1171.

57 Schoendorf KC, et al. Relationship of sudden infant death syndrome to maternal smoking during and after pregnancy. *Pediatrics* 1992;90:905–908.

58 Talor JA, Sanderson MA. Reexamination of the risk factors for the sudden infant death syndrome. *J Pediatr* 1995;126:887–891.

59 Lashner BA, Shaheen NJ, Hanauer SB, Kirschner BS. Passive smoking is associated with an increased risk of developing inflammatory bowel disease in children. *Am J Gastroenterol* 1993;88:356–359.

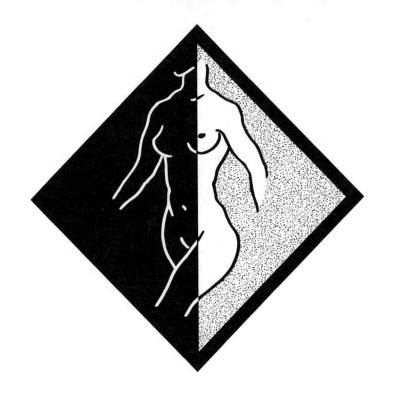

Chapter 10

SMOKING
AND COMPLICATIONS
IN OBSTETRICS AND
GYNECOLOGY

reviewed by
John Patrick O'Grady, M.D.
Director of Obstetrical Services, Chief of Maternal Fetal Medicine,
Professor of Obstetrics and Gynecology,
Baystate Medical Center, Springfield, Massachusetts
Professor of Obstetrics and Gynecology,
Tufts University School of Medicine, Boston, Massachusetts

PART I: COMPLICATIONS OF FERTILITY, PREGNANCY AND NEONATAL HEALTH

The smoking-induced complications experienced by developing and newborn babies are many, and they are potentially of serious consequence. To provide uniform diagnostic criteria for the key features of pregnancy and newborn complications, the term "fetal tobacco syndrome" has been introduced.[1] The very acts of becoming pregnant and maintaining a pregnancy are also much more difficult for smokers than for nonsmokers.

In the first half of this chapter we will review smoking's multiple and serious effects on fertility and pregnancy and will discuss possible mechanisms (when known) for these difficulties. In the second half we will review the gynecological abnormalities other than infertility that women who smoke experience more frequently than nonsmokers.

Infertility

The fertility rates of women who smoke are about 30 percent lower than those of nonsmokers.[2,3] Put another way, smokers are about 3.4 times more likely to take more than a year to conceive than are nonsmokers.[3]

There may be several reasons why women who smoke experience more infertility. Possible reasons include direct damage to the oocytes (eggs) and hormonal irregularities. These hormonal irregularities include abnormal changes in the levels of androgen, follicle-stimulating hormone and estrogen. Female smokers are often said to be estrogen deficient.[4] Smokers' infertility may also be linked to abnormalities in Fallopian tube function. (See the section on smoking and menopause in Part II of this chapter for other consequences of changed estrogen levels.)

Damage to oocytes: Oocytes are the eggs released from a woman's ovaries. Some animal evidence suggests that smoking directly damages or even destroys oocytes, thus impairing fertility.[5]

There is also some evidence that nicotine prevents a protective layer called the *cortical granule* from forming around the oocyte. This layer is designed to prevent additional sperm from penetrating the egg after the first sperm has done so successfully. Scientifically speaking, the cortical granule prevents *polyspermy*. Smokers have more polyspermic embryos (embryos that have been penetrated by many sperm) than do nonsmokers; such embryos fail to develop normally or abort spontaneously. In either case, they may abort very early, leading a woman to count that cycle as one of infertility.[5]

Hormonal irregularities: In women, smoking alters the levels of several hormones, including estrogen and follicle-stimulating hormone. As a result, ovulation (the release of an egg from the ovaries) does not occur normally in smokers, significantly impairing a woman's ability to conceive.[2,5]

Fallopian tube dysfunction: Smoking increases levels of the hormones epinephrine and/or vasopressin, both of which raise blood pressure and heart rate. These normal body chemicals, when produced excessively, may also cause the abnormalities in Fallopian tube function found in women who smoke.

Greater amounts of epinephrine and vasopressin speed up the normal movement of eggs through the Fallopian tubes. These tubes carry the eggs from the ovaries to the uterus; a sperm normally joins with an egg in the Fallopian tube, and the resulting embryo is then transported to the uterus. Some experts theorize that epinephrine and vasopressin cause accelerated propelling waves in the uterus of a smoker, possibly resulting in the early entrance of the embryo into the uterus.

Because timing is so crucial to creating the optimal hormonal milieu conducive to embryo implantation in the uterus, an early entrance of the embryo into the uterus may diminish the possibility that implantation will occur. As a result, the embryo may be lost in a spontaneous abortion.[5] Occurring early, spontaneous abortion is often counted as an infertile cycle.

Paradoxically, in some smokers tubal transport is apparently slowed. This may result in a tubal, or ectopic, pregnancy, or the implantation of the embryo in the Fallopian tube or other site outside the uterus. In a study of 1,108 women with ectopic pregnancies, after controlling for pelvic inflammatory disease and intrauterine device use (both of which increase a woman's risk for ectopic pregnancy), the frequency of this condition was 2.2 to 4 times higher in smokers than in nonsmokers.[6] This is a serious complication of pregnancy that can even cause maternal death if not caught early.

Scientists also theorize that smoking-induced changes in the immune system result in more tubal infections among smokers; this may also explain smokers' greater infertility.[5]

Spontaneous abortions (also called miscarriages): Smokers have been found to have a risk of spontaneous abortion 1.5 to 3.2 times higher than that of nonsmokers.[2,7,8] Tobacco use by pregnant women is responsible for an estimated 19,000 to 141,000 miscarriages each year.[9]

Interestingly, the miscarried fetuses of smoking mothers are much more likely to be chromosomally normal than are those of nonsmokers. This finding supports the hypothesis that smoking impairs a woman's ability to maintain a pregnancy by emphasizing that such miscarriages are not caused by abnormal fetuses,[10] a common cause of miscarriage among nonsmokers.

Limited success of infertility treatment: Not only are smokers more likely to experience infertility, but they are also more likely to have unsuccessful infertility treatments. In particular, smoking patients are much less likely to achieve success with in vitro fertilization and gamete intrafallopian transfer (GIFT) procedures. Also, as with their other pregnancies, smokers who do conceive by such procedures are more likely to suffer miscarriages.[11]

Pregnancy Complications

According to the American College of Obstetrics and Gynecology, carbon monoxide and nicotine are the main ingredients in cigarette smoke responsible for adverse fetal effects.[2]

Adult hemoglobin (the substance in red blood cells that carries oxygen through the bloodstream to tissues) attracts carbon monoxide at a rate 200 times that at which it attracts oxygen. Fetal hemoglobin attracts carbon monoxide at an even greater rate. The carbon monoxide significantly impairs the fetus' ability to bind oxygen, which means that the fetus carried by a smoker experiences significant oxygen deprivation, also known as *hypoxia.*

But smoking deprives the fetus of oxygen by at least two additional mechanisms. Not only does the smoker's hemoglobin bind less oxygen, but it binds oxygen so tightly that less of it can be released to the tissues. The increased levels of epinephrine and other "fight or flight" body chemicals produced in response to the nicotine also decrease blood flow to the fetus.[2]

Smoking has even more far-reaching effects on the fetus than impaired blood flow. Nicotine crosses the placenta (the organ that joins the fetus to the uterus and through which oxygen and nutrients flow to the fetus), raising fetal blood pressure and impairing the fetus' ability to practice breathing motions.[2,12] (The rate at which the fetus has breathing movements is an indication of fetal health.)

The placenta itself is also adversely affected by smoking. Smoking increases a woman's chance of suffering *abruptio placentae* (a condition in which the placenta separates from the uterus too early and which often results in the death of the fetus) and *placenta previa* (a condition in which the placenta attaches to the uterus at an abnormal location, subsequently causing maternal bleeding and possibly fetal death).[2]

The multiple abnormalities experienced by pregnant smokers also result in other problems, including:

Premature rupture of membranes: Smokers are more likely to experience premature rupture of membranes, or their "water breaking" too early.[2] When the fluid-containing sac breaks, a woman can go into labor; this can be very dangerous if the baby is not yet ready to be born. Even if a woman doesn't go into labor, premature rupture of membranes poses a significant problem because it "opens the gate" for bacteria to enter the otherwise sterile environment of the fetus. This can be extremely hazardous for the baby and can result in serious, even life-threatening, infections.

Prematurity: Babies born too early (at fewer than 37 weeks of gestation) face a significantly higher risk of suffering complications and of dying. While estimates vary, the American College of Obstetrics and Gynecology estimates that premature births are 20 percent more common in women who smoke more than one pack per day than in women who don't smoke.[2] Tobacco use by pregnant women is responsible for an estimated 14,000 to 26,000 infants being admitted to neonatal intensive care units each year.[9]

Intrauterine growth retardation and low birth weight: Babies born to mothers who smoke during pregnancy are, on average, about 170 to 200 grams (a quarter to a third of a pound) lighter than those born to nonsmoking mothers.[13,14] Research has shown that these babies are not smaller because they are born early but because they did not develop fully. Technically speaking, such babies are small for gestational age. This may not seem significant, but low birth weight is an important risk factor for neonatal health problems and even for complications later in infancy and childhood.

Cigarette smoking during pregnancy has been recognized as the single most important determinant of poor fetal growth in the developed world. Hypoxia, the lack of oxygen, is an important cause of low birth weight; but other smoking-induced mechanisms are also important. Smoking causes a decreased blood flow to the uterus, a decreased transfer of amino acids (the building blocks of protein) across the placenta to the fetus, abnormalities in the membranes of the placenta and a decreased availability of zinc (a mineral essential to growth).[2,15,16]

Smokers have about a 3.4- to fourfold increase in their chance of having a low birth weight baby. All told, smoking is estimated to account for 21 to 39 percent of all low birth weight babies born in this country.[17] Recently, maternal tobacco use during pregnancy was found to be responsible for an estimated 32,000 to 61,000 low birth weight infants each year.[9] Smoking is one of the strongest risk factors for the most severe form of slow fetal growth: intrauterine growth retardation. Experts deem smoking more important than other factors—including the mother's prepregnancy weight, her height, the number of previous pregnancies, the outcome of her previous pregnancies and infant sex—in causing low birth weight.[17]

Stillbirth: Smokers have an increased risk of delivering stillborn babies. Detailed analyses have revealed that this elevated risk is due to smoking-induced placental complications and smoking-induced intrauterine growth retardation.[18]

Increased risk of transmitting HIV to the fetus: A mother who is HIV positive may pass the infection on to her fetus, and smokers may be more likely to do so. In one study HIV-positive mothers who smoked were 3.3 times as likely to transmit the infection to their fetuses as were nonsmokers.[19]

Birth defects: Until recently, the relationship between smoking and congenital malformations, or birth defects, had been unclear. Overall, maternal smoking had not been shown to be a major risk factor in causing malformations, although some studies had reported a weak association.

One study reported a slight increased risk of 1.6 for congenital malformations among babies whose mothers smoked more than a pack per day during pregnancy as compared with the babies of women who didn't smoke at all.[20] Another study reported a 2.3-fold increase in risk.[21] Interestingly, a 1985 study that looked at the relationship between paternal smoking and birth defects also found an increased rate of congenital malformations.[22]

The first clear-cut association between smoking and a specific birth defect was made in a 1995 study by researchers at Johns Hopkins Children's Center. According to this study babies born to women who smoked during pregnancy had a sixfold increase in cleft palate, the third most common birth defect. This defect is more than cosmetic. Babies with cleft palate—literally a hole in the roof of the mouth—have difficulty swallowing and can even experience difficulty breathing. Some may also have speech problems. The researchers speculated that smoking interferes with the normal action of a gene that controls the proper formation of muscles along the roof of the mouth and the throat.

Does it help if a woman quits smoking immediately upon the confirmation of pregnancy? While it is definitely better for her to stop than to continue, an abnormality such as cleft palate forms in the very earliest days of pregnancy; the damage may already have been done by the time a woman knows she is pregnant.

Maternal well-being: Women who smoke during pregnancy report "feeling awful" much more often than women who don't smoke. According to Jean Golding of the Institutes of Child Health, presenting data from the Avon Longitudinal Study of Pregnancy and Childbirth, smoking mothers rarely experience the feelings of euphoria and well-being that are so common among nonsmokers in the second trimester.[23]

Exposure to passive smoke for at least two hours per day also appears to increase the risk of spontaneous abortion,[24] preterm delivery[24] and low birth weight.[25]

Newborn Complications

Infant allergies: Maternal smoking during pregnancy places offspring at a threefold increased risk of having abnormally high levels of the antibody IgE in the umbilical cord blood at birth. Increased IgE is associated with an increased risk of allergy and places the infant at a fourfold increased risk of having allergic (atopic) skin disease by 18 months of age.[26]

Sudden infant death syndrome: Smoking is also a significant risk factor for sudden infant death syndrome (SIDS), or crib death.[27] Each year tobacco use by pregnant women is responsible for an estimated 1,200 to

2,200 deaths from sudden infant death syndrome.[9] In recent research, Stanford University Medical Center investigators revealed a possible mechanism. Exposure to nicotine, the researchers proposed, may cause an effect similar to jet lag between a mother and her fetus, possibly increasing the risk of SIDS.

In their laboratory work with rats, the Stanford researchers found that nicotine exposure can turn on a gene that influences the biological clock of a fetus while leaving the mother's biological clock unaffected. (The biological clock is a tiny region of the brain that controls daily, or circadian, rhythms, including body temperature and sleep.)

The researchers said that this finding helps scientists understand the development of the brain circuitry that runs the biological clock. The fetal clock is normally entrained by the mother's rhythm, but prenatal exposure to nicotine may interfere with the chemical signals between mother and fetus that bring their clocks into synchrony. The researchers speculated that abnormalities in the infant's circadian timing system could play a role in SIDS and other developmental disorders of the brain.[28]

Perinatal disorders: Each year tobacco use by pregnant women is responsible for an estimated 1,900 to 4,800 infant deaths from disorders occurring around the time of birth.[9]

Intellectual impairment of offspring: The negative effects of maternal smoking during pregnancy continue long after birth. Children of smokers suffer more cognitive and behavioral difficulties[29] and have a decreased ability to achieve in school.[30,31] Some researchers speculate that smoking causes such difficulties because the tobacco by-products released into the bloodstream somehow damage the central nervous system[29]; others hypothesize that smoking-induced hypoxia may play some role in these deficits.[32]

A recent study found maternal smoking during pregnancy to be associated with slightly more than a 50 percent increase in the prevalence of offspring exhibiting unexplained mental retardation and that children whose mothers smoked at least one pack a day during pregnancy had more than a 75 percent increase in the occurrence of unexplained mental retardation.[33]

PART II: COMPLICATIONS IN GYNECOLOGY

Smoking impacts a woman's reproductive system whether or not she is pregnant; serious consequences of smoking commonly appear at menopause. Smoking also increases a woman's risk of cervical cancer (see Chapter 2 for more details). On the other hand, smoking *decreases* a woman's risk of several other conditions. Smoking exerts these effects by reducing the levels of estrogen in a woman's body.

Smoking Leads to Earlier Menopause

While this may seem like good news to some women, an earlier menopause places women at risk for several health problems much earlier than their nonsmoking counterparts. The main reason for earlier menopause among smokers is that smoking lowers estrogen levels in a woman's body. All women experience a gradual diminution in estrogen levels after age 40 and then experience a more rapid decline at menopause. Menstruation stops when a woman no longer produces enough estrogen to maintain the hormonal cycle.

While estrogen withdrawal, as it is known, is a normal part of a woman's life cycle, it has some negative side effects. Most noticeably, estrogen protects a woman against heart disease. This explains why premenopausal women have a lower risk of heart disease than men and why a women's risk increases rapidly to the male level just a few years after menopause.

Estrogen also provides critical protection against osteoporosis, a dangerous thinning of bone that can lead to life-compromising fractures. Smoking compounds this risk. Women who smoke have at least a threefold increased risk of spinal fracture and a twofold increased risk of hip fracture.[34]

According to some estimates, female smokers reach menopause an average of 1.74 years earlier than nonsmokers.[35] Researchers have suggested several possible reasons why this happens. First, nicotine acts on the central nervous system in several ways; some of those actions influence the secretion of hormones involved with menopause. Second, some ingredients of cigarette smoke induce certain liver enzymes that may speed up the breakdown of estrogen.[36,37] This latter mechanism is thought to occur even in women who are not heavy smokers.[38] In women who receive estrogen replacement therapy, smoking increases the rate at which the medication is broken down. Experts do not currently recommend that smokers take higher doses of estrogen to compensate, however.[38]

Other researchers have found that smoking increases the activity of the adrenal gland. The gland then manufacturers greater quantities of androgenic hormones, which further hasten menopause.[37,39]

Yet another hypothesis for the cause of earlier menopause in smokers is that a class of chemicals in cigarette smoke called polycyclic aromatic hydrocarbons destroys eggs (oocytes) in the ovary, thereby bringing on menopause.[34] Smoking may also increase the frequency of the hot flashes so commonly experienced by women in early menopause; this is especially true for thin women.[40]

Protective Effects of Smoking

Further evidence that smoking causes a woman to be estrogen deficient comes from other observations that smokers actually have a lower rate of various conditions influenced by estrogen levels. Women who smoke have less endometrial cancer, fewer uterine fibroids, less endometriosis, less benign breast disease and less *hyperemesis gravidarum* (severe nausea during pregnancy).[34] The harmful effects of cigarette smoking on the female reproductive system and other organ systems far outweigh any of these apparent benefits, however.

References

1   Nieburg P, Marks JS, McLaren NM, Remington PL. The fetal tobacco syndrome. *JAMA* 1985;253:2998–2999.

2   ACOG Technical Bulletin Number 180—May 1990. *Int J Gynecol Obstet* 1993;43:75–81.

3   Baird DD, Wilcox AJ. Cigarette smoking associated with delayed conception. *JAMA* 1985;253:2979–2983.

4   Parazzini F, Ferraroni M, LaVecchia C, et al. Smoking habits and risk of benign breast disease. *Int J Epidemiol* 1991;20:430–434.

5   Stillman RJ, Rosenberg MJ, Sachs BP. Smoking and reproduction. *Fertil Steril* 1986;46:545.

6   Campbell OM, Gray, RH. Smoking and ectopic pregnancy: a multinational case-control study. In Rosenberg MJ, ed. *Smoking and Reproductive Health.* Littleton, Massachusetts: PSG Publishing Co.; 1987:70–75.

7   Gindoff PR, Tidey DF. Effects of smoking on female fecundity and early pregnancy outcome. *Semin Reprod Endocrinol* 1989;7:305–313.

8   Kline J, Stein ZA, Susser M, Warburton D. Smoking: a risk factor for spontaneous abortion. *N Eng J Med* 1977;297:793–796.

9   DiFranza JR, Lew RA. Effect of maternal cigarette smoking on pregnancy complications and sudden infant death syndrome. *J Fam Pract* 1995;40:385–394.

10 Kline J, Levin B, Shrout P, et al. Maternal smoking and trisomy among spontaneously aborted conceptions. *Am J Hum Genet* 1983;35:421–431.

11 Harrison KL, Breen TM, Hennessey JF. The effect of patient smoking habit on the outcome of IVF and GIFT treatment. *Aust NZ J Obstet Gynæcol* 1990;30:340.

12 Manning FA, Feyerabend C. Cigarette smoking and fetal breathing movements. *Br J Obstet Gynæcol* 1976;83:262–270.

13 Sexton M, Hebel JR. A clinical trial of change in maternal smoking and its effect on birth weight. *JAMA* 1984;251:911–915.

14 Spinillo A, Capuzzo E, Nicola SE. Factors potentiating the smoking-related risk of fetal growth retardation. *Br J Obstet Gynæcol* 1994;101:954–958.

15 Harrison KL, Robinson AG. The effect of maternal smoking on carboxyhemoglobin levels and acid-base balance of the fetus. *Clin Toxicol* 1981;18:165–168.

16 Gabriel R, Alsat E, Evain-Brion D. Alteration of epidermal growth factor receptor in placental membranes of smokers: relationship with intrauterine growth retardation. *Am J Obstet Gynecol* 1994;170:1238–1243.

17 U.S. Department of Health and Human Services. *Reducing the Health Consequences of Smoking: 25 Years of Progress.* 1989.

18 Raymond EG, Cnattingius S, Kiely JL. Effects of maternal age, parity, and smoking on the risk of stillbirth. *Br J Obstet Gynæcol* 1994;101:301–306.

19 Burns DN, Landesman S, Muenz LR. Cigarette smoking, premature rupture of membranes, and vertical transmission of HIV-1 among women with low CD4+ levels. *Journal of Acquired Immune Deficiency Syndromes* 1994;7:718–726.

20 Kelsey JL, Dwyer T, Holford TR, Bracken MB. Maternal smoking and congenital malformations: An epidemiological study. *Journal of Epidemiology and Community Health* 1978;32:102–107.

21 Himmelberger DU, Brown BW Jr., Cohen EN. Cigarette smoking during pregnancy and the occurrence of spontaneous abortion and congenital abnormality. *Am J Epidemiol* 1978;108:470–479.

22 Schardein JL. *Chemically Induced Birth Defects.* New York: Marcel Dekker, 1985.

23 Duff E. Smoking and pregnancy conference. *Midwives Chronicle and Nursing Notes* April 1994:128.

24 Ahlborg G, Bodin L. Tobacco smoke exposure and pregnancy outcome among working women. *Am J Epidemiol* 1991;133:338–347.

25 Martin TR, Bracken MB. Association of low birth weight with passive smoke exposure in pregnancy. *Am J Epidemiol* 1986;124:633–642.

26 Magnusson CGM. Maternal smoking influences cord serum IgE and IgE levels and increases the risk for subsequent infant allergy. *J Allergy Clin Immunol* 1986;78:898–904.

27 Rintahaka PJ, Hirvonen J. The epidemiology of sudden infant death syndrome in Finland in 1969–1980. *Forensic Sci Int* 1986;30:219–233.

28 Stanford University Medical Center: *Nicotine Throws Maternal, Fetal Clocks out of Sync.* press release, March 22, 1995.

29 Olds DL, Henderson CR, Tatelbaum R. Intellectual impairment in children of women who smoke cigarettes during pregnancy. *Pediatrics* 1994;93:221–227.

30 Rantakallio P. A follow-up study up to the age of 14 of children whose mothers smoked during pregnancy. *Acta Paediatr Scand* 1983;72:747–753.

31 Naeye RL, Peters EC. Mental development of children whose mothers smoked during pregnancy. *Obstet Gynecol* 1984;64:601–607.

32 Commentary. Cognitive and behavioral abnormalities in children whose mothers smoked cigarettes during pregnancy. *Developmental and Behavioral Pediatrics* 1992;13:425.

33 Drews CD, Murphy CC, Yeargin-Allsopp M, Decoufle P. the relationship between idiopathic mental retardation and maternal smoking during pregnancy. *Pediatrics* 1996;97:547–553.

34 Baron JA, LaVecchia C, Levi F. The antiestrogenic effect of cigarette smoking in women. *Am J Obstet Gynecol* 1990;162:502–514.

35 McKinlay SM, Bifano NL, McKinlay JB. Smoking and age at menopause in women. *Ann Intern Med* 1985;103:350–356.

36 Jick H, Porter J. Relation between smoking and age of natural menopause. *Lancet* June 25, 1977:1354–1355.

37 Cassidenti DL, Pike MC, Vijod AG. A reevaluation of estrogen status in postmenopausal women who smoke. *Am J Obstet Gynecol* 1992;166:1444–1448.

38 Cassidenti DL, Vijod AG, Vijod MA, et al. Short-term effects of smoking on the pharmacokinetic profiles of micronized estradiol in postmenopausal women. *Am J Obstet Gynecol* 1990;163:1953–1960.

39 Schlemmer A, Jensen J, Riis BJ, Christiansen C. Smoking induces increased androgen levels in early post-menopausal women. *Maturitas* 1990;12:99–104.

40 Schwingl PJ, Hulka BS, Harlow SD. Risk factors for menopausal hot flashes. *Obstet Gynecol* 1994;84:29–34.

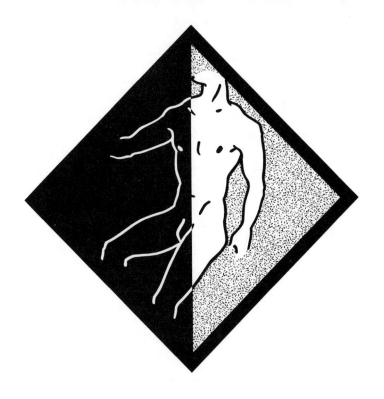

Chapter 11

SMOKING AND UROLOGY: MALE FERTILITY AND SEXUALITY DYSFUNCTIONS

reviewed by
Harris M. Nagler, M.D.
Beth Israel Medical Center, New York, New York
and Albert Einstein College of Medicine
Bronx, New York

The relationship of maternal smoking to fetal harm has long been established. Fewer people are aware, however, that smoking affects a man's reproductive, sexual and urinary organs. The effects may be far-reaching: There is considerable evidence that smoking decreases sperm production, deforms sperm, changes sperm motility (the ability of sperm to move) and seriously reduces blood flow to the penis, in some instances causing impotence.

Not only does smoking affect male reproductive and sexual function, it also causes bladder cancer (see Chapter 2). Smoking has not been determined to increase risk for prostate cancer, but if men with prostate cancer smoke, the smoking appears to cause their cancer to become more invasive and aggressive (see Chapter 2).

How Smoking Affects the Male Reproductive System

Studies have shown that the main metabolites of cigarette smoke (the forms to which inhaled tobacco ingredients are converted in the body) find their way into semen; some of the metabolites even concentrate there.

Levels of cotinine (a by-product of nicotine) and *trans*-3'-hydroxycotinine are found in the semen of smokers at levels similar to the levels at which they are found in the blood. Levels of nicotine found in smokers' semen are even higher than the levels found in their blood, indicating that once absorbed into the bloodstream, nicotine accumulates in seminal fluid.

Components of cigarette smoke that find their way into seminal fluid may contain substances that inhibit a naturally occurring enzyme system, called choline acetyltransferase, that is necessary for sperm to move normally.[1] There is also some evidence that smoking may increase the level of prolactin,[2] a hormone associated with smaller testes[3] and possibly with decreased sperm motility.[3]

Male smokers have lower levels of testosterone[4] (the hormone necessary for sperm production) and higher levels of follicle stimulating hormone[5] (a more feminizing hormone) than do male nonsmokers.

Because of these factors, it appears that cigarette smoking may decrease a man's fertility. Here are some of the specific results of the mechanisms discussed above:

Smoking reduces the amount of ejaculate: Depending on the quantity smoked, smokers ejaculate a decreased volume of semen (with heavier smokers more likely to experience this side effect). Some researchers speculate that this decrease may be caused by nicotine's effect on the nervous system. Smoking may impair the nerves that control the body's ability to ejaculate, thereby causing the decreased volume.[6] There is at least one other mechanism by which ejaculate volume is decreased: Decreased testosterone levels can cause decreased stimulation of the seminal vesicles and result in lower ejaculate volume. While the ejaculate volume per se has little to do with reproductive capacity, it may reflect other abnormalities that can complicate reproduction.

Smoking increases the number of white blood cells in the semen: This complication is called pyospermia; the prefix "pyo" means pus, or infection. In the absence of any detectable sexually transmitted disease (which would be the obvious cause of pyospermia), smokers have a greater incidence of abnormally large numbers of white blood cells in their semen. Because this condition is not associated with a detectable infection, researchers speculate that it is due to smoking-induced inflammation in the reproductive system. The result is that the sperm of a smoker is less able to penetrate the egg *(ovum)*, adversely affecting a couple's ability to conceive.[7]

Smoking impairs sperm count: Extensive evidence now links smoking with decreased sperm count and establishes that smoking directly inhibits the body's ability to produce normal amounts of sperm.[1,8,9,10] Both the cigarette by-products that enter the seminal fluid and the presence of varicocele (an abnormal enlargement of the veins of the spermatic cord) impair sperm quantity. By some estimates, having a varicocele alone raises by tenfold a smoker's chance of having a greatly decreased sperm count.[11] Decreased sperm count is one risk factor for infertility.

Smoking changes the shape of sperm: While not all studies agree, there is considerable evidence that smokers have a higher percentage of sperm with abnormal morphology, or shape.[9,10] This may be related to a greater incidence of miscarriage and congenital malformations, or birth defects.[12]

Smoking impairs sperm motility: Even if normal amounts of sperm are produced (which they aren't in smokers), sperm must move normally for conception to occur. Multiple studies have shown that smokers' sperm do not move normally.[1,8,9,10]

Smoking Is Associated with an Increased Risk of Impotence

Another concern, one difficult for younger smokers to appreciate, is that smoking is a significant risk factor for developing impotence, or the inability to have an erection. One expert has written, "Smoking might have a more deleterious effect on potency than previously anticipated. This information might encourage still-potent men to stop smoking if their sexual desire is stronger than their need of nicotine."[13] While estimates vary, smokers appear to have at least a doubled risk of becoming impotent.[14]

Just as smoking is a significant cause of clogged blood vessels (atherosclerosis) in the heart, it is a critical cause of atherosclerosis in the blood vessels of the penis.[15,16] Because it impairs blood flow, atherosclerosis in the penis is associated with a greatly increased chance of impotence. Impotence that occurs because of impaired blood flow is known as vascular impotence.[17]

In one study of patients at an impotence clinic, 39 percent were diagnosed as having vascular impotence; 97 percent of those men smoked.[18] In another study 82 percent of men with vascular impotence were smokers.[13] The longer a man smokes, the more likely he is to develop vascular impotence. Heavier smoking is also associated with more vascular impotence.[17]

In addition to adversely affecting blood flow to the penis because of atherosclerosis, smoking can lead to impotence because of vasoconstriction (vasoconstriction reduces blood flow because the arteries clamp down).[13,19] Smoking just two cigarettes causes acute vasospasm of the penile arteries.[19] (For more detailed discussion of vasoconstriction, see chapters 3, 7 and 12.)

References

1   Kulikauskas V, Blaustein D, Ablin RJ. Cigarette smoking and its possible effects on sperm. *Fertil Steril* 1985;44:526.

2   Klevene JHH, Balossi EC. Prolactin: a link between smoking and decreased fertility. *Fertil Steril* 1986;46:531.(letter)

3   Sueldo CE, Berger T, Kletzky O, Marrs RP. Seminal prolactin concentration and sperm reproductive capacity. *Fertil Steril* 1985;43:632.

4   Briggs MH. Cigarette smoking and infertility in men. *Med J Aust* 1973;1:616–617.

5   Shaarawy M, Mahmoud KZ. Endocrine profile and semen characteristics in male smokers. *Fertil Sterility* 1982;38:255–257.

6   Marshburn PB, Sloan CS, Hammond MG. Semen quality and association with coffee drinking, cigarette smoking and ethanol consumption. *Fertil Steril* 1989;52:162–165.

7   Close CE, Roberts PL, Berger RE. Cigarettes, alcohol and marijuana are related to pyospermia in infertile men. *J Urol* 1990;144:900–903.

8   Rantala ML, Koskimies AI. Semen quality of infertile couples—comparison between smokers and nonsmokers. *Andrologia* 1986;19:42–46.

9   Vogel W, Broverman DM, Klaiber EL. Gonadal, behavioral and electroencephalograhic correlations of smoking. In: A Remond, C Izard, eds. *Electrophysiological Effects of Nicotine.* Amsterdam: Elsevier-North Holland;1979:201.

10 Evans HJ, Fletcher J, Torrance M, Hargreave TB. Sperm abnormalities and cigarette smoking. *Lancet* 1981;1:627–629.

11 Klaiber EL, Broverman DM, Pokoly, et al. Interrelationships of cigarette smoking, testicular varicoceles and seminal fluid indexes. *Fertil Steril* 1987;47:481.

12 Stillman RJ, Rosenberg MJ, Benjamin P. Smoking and reproduction. *Fertil Steril* 1986;46:554.

13 Forsberg L, Hederstrom E, Olsson AM. Severe arterial insufficiency in impotence confirmed with an improved angiographic technique: the impact of smoking and some other etiologic factors. *Eur Urol* 1989;16:357–360.

14 Mannino DM, Klevens RM, Flander WD. Cigarette smoking: an independent risk factor for impotence. *Am J Epidemiology* 1994;140:1003–1008.

15 Shabsigh R, Rishman IJ, Schum C, Dunn JK. Cigarette smoking and other vascular risk factors in vasculogenic impotence. *Urology* 1991;38:227.

16 Condra M, Morales A, Owen JA, et al. Prevalence and significance of tobacco smoking in impotence. *Urology* 1986;27:495.

17 Rosen MP, Greenfield AJ, Walker TG. Cigarette smoking: an independent risk factor for atherosclerosis in the hypogastric-cavernous arterial bed of men with arteriogenic impotence. *J Impotence* 1991;145:759–763.

18 Bornman MS, DuPlessis DJ. Smoking and vascular impotence: a reason for concern. *S African Med J* 1986;70:329–330.

19 Levine LA, Gerber GS. Acute vasospasm of penile arteries in response to cigarette smoking. *Urology* 1990;36:99.(letter)

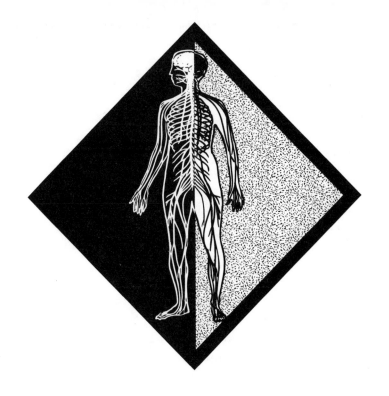

Chapter 12

SMOKING

AND NEUROLOGICAL

DISORDERS

reviewed by
Ognen A.C. Petroff, M.D.
Yale University School
of Medicine

As far back as 1934, researchers knew about nicotine's amazingly potent effect on nerve function. In a laboratory experiment conducted at that time, researchers paralyzed nerves by applying nicotine directly to them.[1]

Today's research into the neurological complications of smoking has produced results that are just as startling. Epidemiological research reveals that over one quarter of strokes—at least 61,500 each year—could be prevented if people stopped smoking. The economic impact of this would be enormous: The total yearly savings could reach $3 billion.[2]

In addition to being one of the two main risk factors for stroke (the other is hypertension), smoking contributes to several other neurological disorders (diseases of the brain and nervous system). Smoking increases the risk for carotid artery disease and transient ischemic attacks (see below for definitions). It also worsens the course of disease in people with multiple sclerosis and other neurological conditions. Moreover, some studies suggest that smoking may impair neuromuscular performance in less obvious ways, so that the risk of subsequent injury is increased.[3] In this chapter we will review the association between smoking and neurological disorders.

Decreased Blood Supply to the Brain

One of the major ways smoking causes neurological problems is by decreasing the blood supply to the brain (also called cerebral blood flow). Smoking has been shown to reduce cerebral blood flow as measured directly in laboratory testing.[4] This reduction is the result of several mechanisms.

As noted in Chapter 3, smoking causes vasoconstriction, or constriction of blood vessels. This constriction causes an immediate reduction in blood flow—in this case, to the brain. Over time, continued vasoconstriction damages the interior of blood vessels. The damaged vessels are more susceptible to accumulating plaque; and once plaque is present in the vessels, continued smoking encourages the progression of the artery-clogging process.

Chronic vasoconstriction also causes blood clots to form on the plaque lesions. If one of these blood clots breaks off and travels to an artery that supplies blood to the brain, it can cause a stroke. Damaged plaque also leads to other problems. As plaque is injured during vasocon-

striction, the lining of blood vessels and blood platelets both release additional substances, leading to even greater vasoconstriction.

In addition to causing vasoconstriction, smoking leads to atherosclerosis. It does this by causing abnormalities in the blood components that impact clotting—both the components that promote clotting and those that keep it in check. Smoking reduces the normal life span of platelets, causing them to clump together abnormally. Smoking also causes platelets to be stickier than normal, again making them more likely to clump. In turn, clumping leads to blood clot formation, which is compounded by smoking's effects on anticlotting factors in the blood. Smoking prevents those factors from dissolving tiny blood clots that continually form in the bloodstream.[5,6,7,8,9,10]

As a result of these many changes, smokers have a greatly increased risk of stroke and transient ischemic attacks (TIAs) as compared with nonsmokers. TIAs are "warning" strokes that can happen before a major stroke—but not everyone who suffers a stroke suffers TIAs first. TIAs occur when a blood clot clogs an artery for a short time. A full-blown stroke happens in one of two ways: Ischemic, or occlusive, strokes occur when the blood supply to the brain is cut off by clots or by totally clogged vessels. Hemorrhagic strokes occur when a blood vessel in the brain bursts. Smoking increases the risk of both types of stroke.[11]

Overall, smokers are two and a half times as likely as nonsmokers to suffer a stroke[12,13]; the risk increases with the number of cigarettes smoked per day. Women who smoke 35 to 44 cigarettes per day are four times as likely to have a stroke as women who have never smoked; the risk rises to 5.4 for women who smoke 45 or more cigarettes per day.[13] Stroke risk has also been quantified by pack-years of smoking. When women who smoke are compared with never smokers, the women with 1 to 9 pack-years of smoking have a 1.7-fold increased risk of stroke; those with 10 to 24 pack-years have a 1.6-fold increased risk. At 25 to 44 pack-years, smokers have a 2.3-fold increased risk; at 45 to 64 pack-years, a 3.1-fold increased risk.[13]

But smoking doesn't just lead to more TIAs and strokes; it also leads to more fatal events[14] and to earlier events.[15] Women under 40 who smoke are at least 2.6 times as likely as nonsmokers to suffer a subarachnoid hemorrhage, a specific type of hemorrhagic stroke.[16,17] Similarly, occlusive stroke, which is very rare in young women, occurs over four times as often in women who smoke as in those who do not.[16]

Finally, the risk of stroke is increased to an even greater extent in smokers who also have other risk factors. For example, patients undergoing heart bypass surgery who have atherosclerosis and/or diabetes are far more likely to suffer a stroke during surgery if they are smokers.[18]

While many people understand that smoking is an important risk factor in causing heart attack, few understand that it also increases their risk of TIA and stroke. Surveys show that consumers are least likely to acknowledge smoking as a risk factor for these disorders.[19]

Fortunately, the increased risk of stroke disappears within two to four years after a person stops smoking.[13] Studies have also shown that cerebral blood flow improves after smoking cessation.[20]

Increased Risk of Carotid Artery Disease

Smokers have a greatly increased risk of carotid artery disease, a blockage in the two main arteries that supply blood to the brain. Blocked carotid arteries, if left untreated, can lead to stroke. Cigarette smoking is the leading risk factor for carotid atherosclerosis in men and is also a significant risk factor for women.

The risk of carotid artery disease increases with increasing pack-years of smoking[21] and remains a significant factor even after controlling for other risk factors for the disease, including high blood pressure and diabetes.[22] Stopping smoking remains one of the most important methods of preventing carotid artery disease and associated stroke.[23]

Worsened Symptoms in Patients with Multiple Sclerosis

Smoking has been associated with a temporary worsening of symptoms of multiple sclerosis. Most notably, patients' upper-body motor functioning deteriorates with smoking.[24,25] Other symptoms that worsen with smoking include tremor, leg weakness, spasticity, loss of sensation in the extremities, incoordination, trouble walking and visual disturbances.[24]

The mechanism by which smoking worsens motor functioning in multiple sclerosis is uncertain, but researchers offer several theories, most of them based on nicotine acting as a potent toxin to the central nervous system. Included among the possible mechanisms are the following:[24]

- Nicotine disrupts nerve function; in particular, smoking disrupts the nerves that control involuntary movements.

- Nicotine interferes with nerve-muscle communication; it may act on the sites where nerves communicate with muscles to tell them what to do.

- Smoking decreases cerebral blood flow. While all smokers suffer decreased cerebral blood flow, the reduced flow poses even more problems to the already-damaged nerve cells of patients with multiple sclerosis and thereby worsens the symptoms of multiple sclerosis.

- Smoking decreases oxygen levels in the blood. Again, while this occurs in all smokers, it poses even more of a problem for the already damaged nerve cells in people with multiple sclerosis.

- Nicotine causes abnormalities in blood vessels; in turn, these vascular abnormalities impair motor functioning in multiple sclerosis patients.

Smoking May Worsen Other Neurological Conditions

Although reports on the subject are anecdotal and have not involved controlled studies, it appears that smoking may also worsen other neurological diseases. In particular, smoking worsens symptoms in patients with multiple system atrophy,[26] a disorder in which the autonomic nervous system (the nerves that control automatic body functions such as blood pressure, bowel and bladder functions and sweating) does not function properly. This leads to multiple and serious problems.

The association between reflex sympathetic dystrophy and smoking has been studied to only a limited degree, but there is some suggestion that smoking plays a role in causing this painful disorder or at least has a role in worsening it.[27] Reflex sympathetic dystrophy is a painful, chronic neurological condition in which one type of nerve cell dysfunctions to cause intense pain, abnormal sweating and other problems. Commonly, this condition develops in an extremity after an injury, but there can be many other precipitating factors, including infection and arthritis.

Smoking also appears to worsen spinocerebellar degeneration,[28] a complex neurological disorder that leads to spinal cord dysfunction. Brain dysfunction caused by excess alcohol consumption is also worsened by smoking.[29] Other reports link smoking with a worsening of Shy-Drager syndrome, another serious neurological disorder in which the autonomic nervous system does not function properly.[30,31]

Smoking Alters the Energy-Controlling Mechanism of the Body

In laboratory experiments, smoking has been shown to interact with the mitochondria, the portions of cells that play a significant role in energy metabolism. Researchers have noted further that smoking affects mitochondrial disorders, complex neurological diseases that are mediated by defects of metabolism involving the mitochondria.[32]

Protection from Some Neurological Disorders

That smoking has powerful effects on the nervous system is emphasized by the fact that it seems to afford protection against Parkinson's disease and Alzheimer's disease.

While research results aren't conclusive, there are several possibilities to explain smoking's protective effect against Parkinson's disease. Parkinson's disease occurs because of a relative deficiency of dopamine, a neurotransmitter. Among many other critical jobs, dopamine is necessary in certain quantities to ensure the smooth processing of the "orders" the brain gives to muscles to tell them when and how to move. Nicotine may correct the abnormality that leads to the symptoms of Parkinson's; specifically, nicotine may restore dopamine to normal levels.[33,34]

Another possible mechanism is that smoking stimulates the production of certain cells in the mouth—melanocytes—that are thought to bind and render inactive toxic substances known to worsen symptoms in Parkinson's disease.[35]

While the detrimental effects of cigarette smoking far outweigh any possible protective effect of smoking against Parkinson's disease, this association contributes to our understanding of the underlying nature of Parkinson's disease and how to treat it. [36]

The risk of Alzheimer's disease appears to decrease with increasing numbers of cigarettes smoked per day and increasing pack-years of smoking.[37] One possible mechanism by which smoking protects against Alzheimer's disease is by boosting the function of the neurotransmitter acetylcholine.[38] Other researchers postulate, however, that the gene pool of smokers and nonsmokers is different and that it is actually the difference in genes associated with Alzheimer's disease that accounts for the paradox, rather than any protective effect of smoking.[39]

As with Parkinson's disease, experts note that the advantage of preventing Alzheimer's disease by smoking is far outweighed by the well-documented risks to smokers of developing chronic conditions such as cancer and cardiovascular disease.[37]

References

1   Haggard HW, Greenberg L. The effects of cigarette smoking upon the blood sugar. *Science* 1934;79:165–166.

2   Gorelick P. Stroke prevention: an opportunity for efficient utilization of health care resources during the coming decade. *Stroke* 1994;25:220–224.

3   Slade J. Smoking, alcohol, and neuromuscular function in older women (letter). *JAMA* 1995;273:1333-1334.

4   Mathew R, Wilson W. Substance abuse and cerebral blood flow. *Am J Psychiatry* 1991;148:292–305.

5   Higa M, Davanipour Z. Smoking and stroke. *Neuroepidemiology* 991;10:211–222.

6   Wilhelmsen L, Svardsudd K, Korsan-Bengsten K, et al. Fibrinogen as a risk factor for stroke and myocardial infarction. *N Engl J Med* 1984;311:501–505.

7   Mehta P, Mehta J. Effects of smoking on platelets and on plasma thromboxane-prostacyclin balance in man. *Prostaglandins Leukotrienes Me* 1982;9:141–150.

8   Dintefass L. Elevation of blood viscosity, aggregation of red cells, hæmatocrit values and fibrinogen levels in cigarette smokers. *Med J Aust* 1975;i:617–620.

9   Rogers RL, Meyer JS, Shaw TG, et al. Cigarette smoking decreases cerebral blood flow suggesting increased risk for stroke. *JAMA* 1983;250:2796–2800.

10 McGill HC. Potential mechanism for the augmentation of atherosclerosis and atherosclerotic disease by cigarette smoking. *Prevent Med* 1979;8:390–403.

11 Abbott RD, Yin Y, Reed DM Yano K. Risk of stroke in male cigarette smokers. *N Engl J Med* 1986;315:717–720.

12 Robbins A, Manson J, Lee M, et al. Cigarette smoking and stroke in a cohort of U.S. male physicians. *Ann Intern Med* 1994;120:458–462.

13 Kawachi I, Colditz G, Stampfer M, et al. Smoking cessation and decreased risk of stroke in women. *JAMA* 1993;269:232–236.

14 Haheim L, Holme I, Leren P. Risk factors of stroke incidence and mortality: a 12-year followup of the Oslo study. *Stroke* 1993;24:1484–1489.

15 Giovannoni G, Fritz VU. Transient ischemic attacks in younger and older patients. *Stroke* 1993;24:947–953.

16 Thorogood M, Mann J, Murphy M, Vessey M. Fatal stroke and use of oral contraceptives: findings from a case-control study. *Am J Epidemiol* 1992; 136:35–45.

17 Shinton R, Beevers G. Meta-analysis of relationship between cigarette smoking and stroke. *Br Med J* 1989;298:789–794.

18 Lynn G, Stefanko K, Reed J, et al. Risk factors for stroke after coronary bypass. *J Thorac Cardiovasc Surg* 1992;104:1518–1523.

19 Desmond D, Tatemichi T, Paik M, Stern Y. Risk factors for cerebrovascular disease as correlates of cognitive function in a stroke-free cohort. *Arch Neurol* 1993;50:162–166.

20 Gorelick P, Brody J, Cohen D, et al. Risk factors for dementia associated with multiple cerebral infarcts: a case-control analysis in predominantly African-American hospital-based patients. *Arch Neurol* 1993;50:714–720.

21 Willeit J, Keichl S. Prevalence and risk factors of asymptomatic extracranial carotid artery atherosclerosis: a population-based study. *Arteriosclerosis and Thrombosis* 1993;13:661–668.

22 Dempsey R, Moore R. Amount of smoking independently predicts carotid artery atherosclerosis severity. *Stroke* 1992;23:693–696.

23 Barnett H. Therapy of carotid arteriosclerosis. *Ann Rev Med* 1994;45:53–69.

24 Emre M, de Decker C. Effects of cigarette smoking on motor functions in patients with multiple sclerosis. *Arch Neurol* 1992;49:1243–1247.

25 Courville CB, Maschmeyer JE, Delay CP. Effect of smoking on the acute exacerbations of multiple sclerosis. *Bulletin of the Los Angeles Neurological Society* 1964;29:1.

26 Johnsen JA, Miller VT. Tobacco intolerance in multiple system atrophy. *Neurology* 1986;36:986–988.

27 An HS, Hawthorne KB, Jackson TW. Reflex sympathetic dystrophy and cigarette smoking. *J Hand Surg* 1988;13A:458–460.

28 Spillane JD. The effect of nicotine on spinocerebellar ataxia. *Br Med J* 1955;2:1345–1351.

29 Schitt J, Seelinger D, Appenzeller O, Orrison W. Nicotine and alcoholic cerebellar degeneration. *Neurology* 1988;38(suppl 1):205. Abstract.

30 Johnson RH, De JG, Oppenheimer DR, et al. Autonomic failure with orthostatic hypotension due to intermediolateral column degeneration. A report of two cases with autopsies. *Quarterly Journal of Medicine* 1966;35:276.

31 Graham GH, Oppenheimer DR. Orthostatic hypotension and nicotine sensitivity in a case of multiple system atrophy. *Journal of Neurology, Neurosurgery and Psychiatry* 1969;32:28.

32 Smith P. Cooper J. Govan G. Smoking and mitochondrial function: a model for environmental toxins. *Quarterly Journal of Medicine* 1993;86:657–660.

33 Jarvik M. Beneficial effects of nicotine. *British Journal of Addiction* 1991;86:571–575.

34 Ishikawa A. Effects of smoking in patients with early-onset Parkinson's disease. *Journal of the Neurological Sciences* 1993;117:28–32.

35 Hedin CA. Smoker's melanosis may explain the lower hearing loss and lower frequency of Parkinson's disease found among tobacco smokers—a new hypothesis. *Medical Hypotheses* 1991;35:247–249.

36 Grandinetti A., Morens D, Reed D, MacEachern D. Prospective study of cigarette smoking and the risk of developing idiopathic Parkinson's disease. *Am J Epidemiol* 1994;139:1129–1138.

37 Rocca W. Frequency, distribution and risk factors for Alzheimer's disease. *Nurs Clin North Am* 1994;29:101–111.

38 Jones G, Sahakian B, Warburton D, Gray J. Effects of acute subcutaneous nicotine on attention, information processing and short-term memory in Alzheimer's disease. *Pscyhopharmacology* 1992;108:485–494.

39 Hardy J, Roberts G. Smoking and neurogenerative diseases. *Lancet* 1993;342:1238.

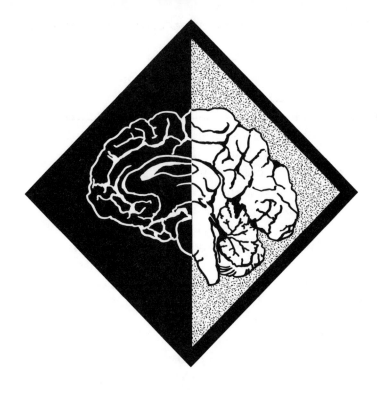

Chapter 13

PSYCHIATRY:

SMOKING, THE BRAIN

AND BEHAVIOR

reviewed by
Glenn Swogger, Jr., M.D.
Senior Psychiatric Consultant (retired)
The Menninger Management Institute
Topeka, Kansas

Ancient populations used tobacco for both medicinal and recreational purposes.[1] The primary psychoactive drug in tobacco, nicotine, causes rapid and multiple physiological effects. When cigarette smoke is inhaled, the nicotine first stimulates sensory nerve endings embedded in the vicinity of the millions of air sacs of the lungs. Within seconds this stimulation produces a powerful reflex effect consisting of a brief, abrupt fall in heart rate and blood pressure (soon followed by opposite effects); a generalized relaxation of the body musculature; and a simultaneous arousal of the brain.[2] The combination of physical relaxation and comfort with mental alertness is the unique characteristic of nicotine and is responsible for the instantaneous "rush" that the smoker feels and seeks. Indeed, the first changes in electroencephalogram (EEG) readings—which measure the electrical activity in the brain—occur before nicotine reaches the brain. Both muscle relaxation and EEG arousal are then reinforced by nicotine action on neuronal circuits in brain and spinal cord.

In this chapter, we'll review how smoking affects the brain and the smoker's ability to perform mental tasks. We'll also review the association between smoking and depression and the relationship between smoking and other psychiatric disorders.

How Smoking Affects the Brain

The brain is often referred to as a very "privileged" area. Its internal milieu is protected from unwelcome changes by a remarkably thin layer of tissue, the blood-brain barrier. Although the blood-brain barrier effectively blocks most substances from entering the brain, nicotine rapidly crosses it. Once across, the nicotine quickly causes several changes.

Within 10 seconds of the first inhalation, nicotine slips easily past the blood-brain barrier and begins to act on a specific set of neurons, the working cells of the brain. On each of these neurons are receptors, which are much like slots or keyholes onto which brain chemicals called neurotransmitters attach, causing the brain to transmit messages. Nicotine fits into one of the receptors acted upon by acetylcholine, one of several neurotransmitters in the brain.

Normally, when acetylcholine attaches to the receptors, it triggers the nerve cells to communicate with each other so that the brain can "tell" other parts of the body what to do (nerve cells must communicate, for example, when the brain wants to tell the hand to pick up a cup of coffee). When nicotine slides into these receptors, however, it triggers quite a different reaction: It causes the brain to release two other substances, noradrenaline and dopamine, that act as stimulants.

How Smoking Affects Cognitive Function

Many smokers believe that smoking improves cognition, or the ability to perform mental tasks. Very often, a smoker will light up repeatedly in an attempt to remain sharp while performing mental work or to cope with the demands of life. One proposed explanation is that nicotine-dependent smokers light up to avoid the symptoms of withdrawal. However, even in the absence of nicotine dependence, smoking increases alertness, cognitive performance and the ability to sustain performance while fatigued.[3]

Smoking and Depression

Depression—whether viewed as a trait, a symptom or a diagnosable disorder—is overrepresented among smokers.[4,5]

Depression and cigarette smoking are intertwined in a manner that is complex and not well understood. People who are depressed are more likely to smoke; smokers are more likely to be depressed; and depressed smokers have a more difficult time managing their depression if they try to stop smoking. In addition, smokers with a history of depression have more intense psychologic symptoms; and these depressive symptoms are magnified to an even greater degree when these people try to stop smoking.[6] In this complicated symbiosis of smoking and depression, researchers remain uncertain as to which is the driving force: the smoking or the depression.[7]

Some of the issues that researchers speculate may be at play in the smoking-depression picture are the following:[6]

- Smoking—and, in particular, nicotine—may have a direct depressant effect.

- Smokers may have poor self-image because of the stigma associated with smoking.

- Smokers may become troubled because although they know smoking will eventually damage their health, they are unable to stop smoking.

- Smokers may develop a chronic illness because of smoking, and the chronic illness they suffer may have a depressant effect.

- Smokers may be self-medicating their depression and/or anxiety with cigarettes.

- Smokers may have some genetic or environmental predisposition to developing depression.

Not only are depressed smokers (as compared with nondepressed smokers) more likely to experience withdrawal symptoms when they attempt to quit, but they are also less likely to be successful at quitting and more likely to relapse. In one large study of smoking cessation, depression was the most significant reason for relapse. The authors of the study estimated that 30 to 40 percent of adults who begin smoking-cessation programs are depressed—that's *three times* the rate of depression in nonsmokers. The researchers called for smoking-cessation programs to be specially tailored to the needs of depressed smokers.[8]

Other researchers have found that antidepressant therapy, psychological support and nicotine-replacement therapy are all useful adjuncts in helping the depressed smoker to quit.[5]

Smoking and Other Psychiatric Disorders

The proportion of smokers among psychiatric patients is considerably higher than the proportion of adults who currently smoke in the general population. The most common psychiatric disorder noted among smokers is schizophrenia.[9] In one study 74 percent of schizophrenic patients smoked; overall, about 25 percent of the general population smokes.[7] Most likely this means that smoking is appealing to schizophrenics, and not that smoking leads to schizophrenia. Smoking rates are also high among alcoholics, among agoraphobics (people abnormally fearful of open places) and among those with panic disorder and other anxiety conditions. Although many people with anxiety smoke to relieve those symptoms, the anxiety-depleting effects of smoking have been difficult to replicate in studies.[7]

Interestingly, while there is a trend today toward smoke-free hospitals, smoke-filled psychiatric wards and chemical dependency treatment centers still abound. Furthermore, patients and their advocates strongly resist institutional restrictions on smoking. Even psychiatric experts are uncertain of the association: Do psychiatric patients treat their symptoms by smoking, or do they smoke to alleviate the side effects of medication? Do they start smoking for one of these reasons and then develop a tolerance?[9] Some studies have found that smoking may actually worsen psychiatric disorders, cloud and confuse treatment and even impair long-term prognoses.[10] Further research is clearly needed to clarify this association.

References

1   Le Houezec J, Benowitz NL. Basic and clinical psychopharmacology of nicotine. *Smoking Cessation* 1991;12:681–699.

2   Ginzel KH. The lungs as the site of origin of nicotine-induced skeletomotor relaxation and behavioral and EEG arousal in the cat. In: Rand MD and Thurau K, eds. *The Pharmacology of Nicotine.* Satellite Symposium of the 10th International Congress of Pharmacology, Golcoast, Queensland, Australia, 1987. Publishing House of the International Council of Scientific Unions Symposium Series, Vol. 9.: ICSU Press; 1988: 269–292.

3   Glassman AH. Psychoactive smoke. *Nature* 1996; 37:677–678.

4   Glass RM. Blue mood, blackened lungs. *JAMA* 1990; 264:153–1584.

5   Hall S, Munoz R, Reus V, Sees K. Nicotine, negative affect and depression. *Journal of Consulting and Clinical Psychology* 1993;61:761–767.

6   Frank SH, Jaen CR. Office evaluation and treatment of the dependent smoker. *Substance Abuse* 1993;20:251–268.

7   Glassman A. Cigarette smoking and implications for psychiatric illness. *Am J Psychiatry* 1993;150:4:546–553.

8   Lerman C, Audrain J, Orleans T, et al. Investigation of mechanisms linking depressed mood to nicotine dependence. *Addictive Behavior* 1996;21(1):9–19.

9   Kirch D. Where there's smoke . . . nicotine and psychiatric disorders. Editorial. *Biol Psychiatry* 1991;30:107–108.

10 Newhouse P, Hughes J. The role of nicotine and nicotinic mechanisms in neuropsychiatric disease. *Br J Addiction* 1991;86:521–526.

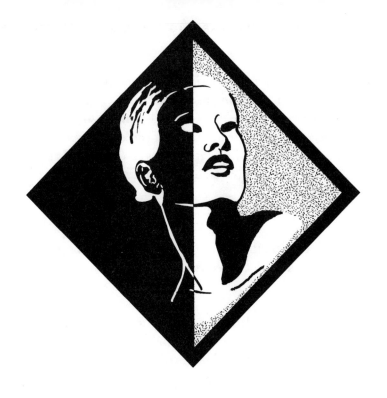

Chapter 14

OTOLARYNGOLOGY: ABNORMALITIES OF THE EARS, NOSE AND THROAT ASSOCIATED WITH SMOKING

reviewed by
David R. Nielsen, M.D.
Southwest Otologic Institute, Ltd.
Phoenix, Arizona

Smoking is associated with a variety of abnormalities in the ears, nose and throat, including hearing loss and snoring. In this chapter we will review the evidence for smoking-induced abnormalities in conditions treated by otolaryngologists (ear, nose and throat specialists). For related information on ear, nose and throat diseases in children that are associated with environmental tobacco smoke or passive smoking, please refer to Chapter 9.

Snoring

People who smoke more than 15 cigarettes per day are six and a half times as likely as nonsmokers to be frequent snorers.[1]

Hearing Loss

Smokers have an increased risk of several types of hearing loss: sudden hearing loss; hearing loss associated with chronic exposure to loud noise; hearing loss associated with middle-ear fluid and infection (see Chapter 9); and acceleration of the hearing loss associated with aging.

Smokers experience sudden hearing loss an average of 16 years earlier than do never smokers. In addition, smokers are more likely than nonsmokers to experience recurrent sudden hearing loss: 46 percent of smokers suffer such a recurrence, while just 33 percent of nonsmokers do.[2]

Noise is the most common hazardous exposure in the workplace; at any given time, nearly eight million U.S. workers are exposed to noises that are too loud. There is great variation in how people respond to excessive noise; some experience noise-induced hearing loss and others do not. The reasons for this variability remain unidentified.

Smoking is one factor known to increase a person's chance of suffering noise-induced hearing loss. Both total smoking exposure (as measured by pack-year history) and intensity of present smoking (as measured by packs per day) correlate directly with loss of hearing brought about by chronic exposure to excessively loud noise.[3]

While experts aren't entirely sure how smoking increases a person's risk of hearing loss caused by chronic exposure to loud noise, they believe smoking-induced decreased blood flow to the ears plays a role. The inner ear contains the sensory cells and other tissues critical to hearing, and the vessels that carry blood to the inner ear can become blocked by atherosclerosis. Loud noise further compromises blood flow to the inner ear because the body responds to loud noises with vasoconstriction, cutting off the blood supply to the inner ear. Finally, some researchers believe that high levels of carbon monoxide in the blood of smokers may directly damage sensory cells in the inner ear.[3]

Hearing loss directly related to aging is called presbyacusis. While this type of hearing loss is common, there is some evidence that smoking may accelerate it.[4]

Dizziness

Smoking, especially among the uninitiated, may cause dizziness. This is due, at least in part, to a disturbance of the vestibular apparatus, a part of the inner ear that plays an important role in balance.[2]

Nasal Congestion

People with chronic rhinitis (a chronic inflammation of the nose) suffer sneezing, nasal congestion and a runny and itchy nose. While most experts agree that smoking worsens chronic rhinitis or possibly even causes it, there is little supporting documentation to solidify the association. Solidifying the relationship between smoking and chronic rhinitis is difficult because the condition has so many causes and associations.[5]

References

1 Stradling JR, Crosby JH. Predictors and prevalence of obstructive sleep apnœa and snoring in 1001 middle aged men. *Thorax* 1991;46:85–90.

2 Matschke RG. Smoking habits in patients with sudden hearing loss. *Acta Otolaryngol* (Stockh) 1991;476(suppl):69–73.

3 Barone JA, Peters JM, Garabrant DH, et al. Smoking as a risk factor in noise-induced hearing loss. *Journal of Occupational Medicine* 1987;29:741–745.

4 Rosenhall U, Sixt E, Sundh V, Svanborg A. Correlations between presbyacusis and extrinsic noxious factors. *Audiology* 1993;32:234–243.

5 Small P, Barrett D. Nonspecific nasal reactivity and smoking. *Annals of Allergy* 1994;73:114–116.

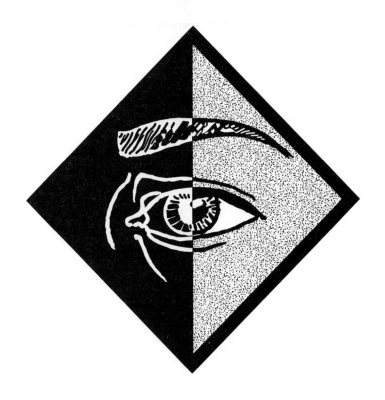

Chapter 15

SMOKING
AND THE EYES

reviewed by
Emil W. Chynn, M.D.
Emory University Department of Ophthalmology
Atlanta, Georgia
and Frederick L. Ferris, M.D.
National Eye Institute

Many nonsmokers are acutely aware of the irritating effects smoking has on their eyes; they suffer burning, watering and reddened eyes in the presence of cigarette smoke. Few smokers, however, are aware of the many—and serious—eye diseases they may suffer as a result of their smoking. Smoking can cause or worsen over half a dozen eye conditions, some of which can lead to permanent vision loss.

In this chapter we will describe the eye diseases suffered by smokers and, when known, explain the possible mechanisms that account for them.

Smoking and Cataracts

At least 50 million people around the world lose vision as a result of cataracts. In the United States alone, cataracts annually claim at least part of the vision of 3.3 million people. When a cataract develops, it causes a loss of transparency in the eye's lens. This translates into a gradual, painless loss of vision. When cataracts are detected early, they can be removed surgically and vision can be restored.

While cataracts can develop as a result of the normal aging process, certain risk factors increase the likelihood of their developing. Having diabetes and taking certain medications—corticosteroids, for example—both increase the chance that a person will develop cataracts. Smoking is another potent risk factor for cataracts. Compared with never smokers, current smokers of 20 or more cigarettes per day are at least twice as likely to develop any type of cataract and three times as likely to develop a particular type of cataract called posterior subcapsular cataract. This type of cataract is especially visually disabling.[1,2]

The smoker's risk of cataract increases with the amount smoked; in addition, cataracts are more serious in heavy smokers than in light smokers.[3] Finally, former smokers continue to have a 50 percent increased risk for cataract.[1]

Researchers remain uncertain as to whether cataracts develop as a result of external irritation from cigarette smoke; as a result of the biochemical effect of some constituent of smoke that is absorbed via the lungs and subsequently travels to the eye via the bloodstream; or as a result of some combination of the two.[4]

Of the many proposed mechanisms for the smoking–cataract association, the destruction of antioxidant nutrients and subsequent increased formation of oxidative-free radicals are leading contenders. Among their many other jobs, antioxidants play a critical role in maintaining lens transparency by preventing direct oxidation of lens proteins. They also prevent lipid peroxidation, a process that causes the breakdown of the fatty membranes that make up the lens of the eye.[4] Cigarette smoking may also break down other micronutrients critical to healthy eye tissue.[1]

Some researchers speculate, in yet another theory, that the metallic element cadmium found in cigarette smoke (tobacco leaves absorb and concentrate cadmium from the soil) plays a role in cataract development. It is possible that the cadmium binds with and damages the proteins in the lens.[5]

Smoking and Graves' Disease

In Graves' disease, the thyroid gland becomes overactive, secreting too much thyroid hormone. Many sites of the body suffer negative effects, but eye complications are the most serious consequence of the disorder.[6] Excess hormone can cause protrusion of the eyes, double vision, eye-muscle abnormalities and even permanent blindness.

When Graves' patients smoke, they have a nearly eightfold-increased risk of developing the eye complications as compared with nonsmoking Graves' patients.[7] In addition, the smokers suffer the eye symptoms in a more severe form.[6,8]

The reason for smokers' increased risk of eye involvement in Graves' disease remains uncertain, but it may be due to a smoking-induced impairment of the immune system. Smoking changes the number of T cells produced in the immune system; it also causes the body to produce other types of cells that trigger inflammatory reactions in various sites in the body, including the eye.[9] Because Graves' disease is, in fact, a disorder of the immune system, these latter possibilities are plausible. (See Chapter 19 for more detail on the components of the immune system.)

Smoking and Age-Related Macular Degeneration

Macular degeneration is damage to or breakdown of the macula, the small central area of the retina at the back of the eye that allows people to see fine details clearly. When the macula doesn't function correctly, vision becomes blurred and dark in the center; peripheral vision is generally not affected. Macular degeneration is the leading cause of blindness in adults over 65.

There is no treatment to prevent this serious condition, but there is one very controllable risk factor: smoking. Women who smoke appear to have about a 2.5-fold increase in risk of developing one form of macular degeneration—exudative macular degeneration, a more severe form of the disease that results in a more rapid and severe loss of vision. Men who smoke appear to have more than a threefold increased risk.[10] In exudative macular degeneration, abnormal blood vessels form at the back of the eye. These new blood vessels leak fluid or blood and blur central vision. Smokers appear to be more likely to suffer this more severe form of macular degeneration[11] and to suffer relapse after palliative laser treatment.[12]

Smoking and Ocular Histoplasmosis Syndrome

Ocular histoplasmosis syndrome, an inflammation of the eye thought to be caused by a fungus commonly found in soil, is also associated with smoking: Heavy smokers suffer far more ocular histoplasmosis syndrome than do people who don't smoke.[13]

Smoking and Abnormal Eye Movements

Smoking may cause nystagmus, or abnormal eye movements. These movements can include jerking and/or rhythmical oscillations (circular movements). The ingredient in cigarette smoke responsible for this hasn't been identified, but nicotine remains the most likely candidate. Nicotine may possibly cause nystagmus by disrupting the balance center (called the vestibular apparatus) of the brain.[14]

Smoking and Diabetic Retinopathy

Smoking may accelerate the development of or worsen an eye complication associated with diabetes, diabetic retinopathy. In this disease, which can lead to blindness, the vessels that supply blood to the retina (a nerve layer at the back of the eye that senses light and helps send messages to the brain) are damaged by repeated high blood sugars. When these blood vessels become damaged, they may leak fluid or blood and grow scar tissue. Both the leaking of fluid and the growth of scar tissue can distort the images the retina sends to the brain.

It is plausible that smoking worsens this condition because it, too, damages blood vessels (see chapters 3 and 4). A possible mechanism leading to damage to the blood vessels of the eyes is smoking-induced hypoxia. This condition is a result of diminished oxygen in the blood, with a corresponding increase in carbon monoxide levels. Experts warn that low-nicotine cigarettes are not an answer, as their smoke actually contains a larger amount of carbon monoxide than does smoke from higher nicotine cigarettes.[15]

Smoking and Optic Neuropathy

Anterior ischemic optic neuropathy is an eye disease that results in a sudden, painless loss of vision, often leading to permanent blindness. It occurs because of compromised blood flow, or even a total lack of blood flow, in specific arteries that supply the eyes. Experts believe that atherosclerosis—the clogging of arteries—in the optic area may play a role in causing this disease.

It has recently been discovered that smoking is a significant risk factor for developing this serious eye disease. Smokers are at a 16-fold increased risk of developing anterior ischemic optic neuropathy as compared with nonsmokers.[16] In addition, smokers develop the disorder at younger ages; in one study smokers were found to develop the disease at an average age of 51 and nonsmokers at an average age of 64.[17]

Smoking and Optic Neuritis

The optic nerve carries messages from the eye to the brain. This nerve critical to vision is like a cable of electrical wires; it consists of about 1.2 million separate tiny nerve fibers, each of which is a conduit for part of the brain's message. Vision is not normal unless the overwhelming majority of these tiny fibers work properly and are healthy. In optic neuritis, the optic nerve becomes inflamed, or swollen and red. When a significant number of the tiny fibers in the optic nerve become inflamed, vision may be affected. People who suffer from optic neuritis may have pain, blurred vision and/or a blind spot in their vision.

Smokers with optic neuritis are far more likely to develop an additional defect: specifically, a red/green color defect in the affected eye. While experts are not sure of the mechanism for this, they propose that the red/green defect occurs because of the relative lack of oxygen reaching the eye in smokers as compared with nonsmokers.[18]

Tobacco Amblyopia

Smoking may result in tobacco amblyopia, or a loss of vision in both eyes. For many years experts thought this rare condition could occur only if malnutrition, alcoholism or a disorder of vitamin B_{12} metabolism also existed. Two fairly recent case reports, however, have suggested that tobacco amblyopia can occur independent of these other conditions. Cessation of smoking can result in a total cure.[19]

References

1   Christen WG, Manson JE, Seddon JM, et al. A prospective study of cigarette smoking and risk of cataract in men. *JAMA* 1992;268:989–993.

2   Flaye DE, Sullivan KN, Cullinan TR, et al. Cataracts and cigarette smoking. *Eye* 1989;3:379–384.

3   West S, Munoz B, Emmett E, Taylor HR. Cigarette smoking and risk of nuclear cataracts. *Arch Ophthalmol* 1989;107:1166–1169.

4   Hankinson SE, Willett WC, Colditz GA, et al. A prospective study of cigarette smoking and risk of cataract surgery in women. *JAMA* 1992;268:994–998.

5   Ramakrishnan S, Sulochana KH, Selvaraj T, et al. Smoking of beedies and cataract: cadmium and vitamin C in the lens and blood. *Br J Ophthalmol* 1995;79:202–206.

6   Winsa B, Mandahl A, Karlsson FA. Graves' disease, endocrine ophthalmopathy and smoking. *Acta Endocrinologica* 1993;128:156–160.

7   Prummel MF, Wieringa WM. Smoking and risk of Graves' disease. *JAMA* 1993;269:479–482.

8   Hagg E, Asplung K. Is endocrine ophthalmopathy related to smoking? *Br Med J* 1987;295:634–635.

9   Shine B, Fells P, Edwards OM, Weetman AP. Association between Graves' ophthalmopathy and smoking. *Lancet* 1990;335:1261–1263.

10 Klein R, Klein BEK, Linton KLP, DeMets DL. The Beaver Dam Eye Study: the relation of age-related maculopathy to smoking. *Am J Epidemiol* 1993;137:190–200.

11 Paetkau ME, Boyd TAS, Grace M, et al. Senile disciform macular degeneration and smoking. *Can J Ophthalmol* 1978;13:67–71.

12 Macular Photocoagulation Study Group. Recurrent choroidal neovascularization after argon laser photocoagulation for neovascular maculopathy. *Arch Ophthalmol* 1986;104:503–512.

13 Ganley JP. Epidemiologic characteristics of presumed ocular histoplasmosis. *Acta Ophthalmol* Suppl (Copenh) 1973;119:1–63.

14 Sibony PA, Evinger C, Manning KA. Tobacco-induced primary-position upbeat nystagmus. *Ann Neurol* 1987;21:53–58.

15 Paetkau ME. Diabetic retinopathy and smoking. *Lancet* Nov. 18, 1978:1098–1099.

16 Talks SJ, Chong NHV, Gibson JM, Dodson PM. Fibrinogen, cholesterol and smoking as risk factors for non-arteritic anterior ischæmic optic neuropathy. *Eye* 1995;9:85–88.

17 Chung SM, Gay CA, McCrary JA. Nonarteritic ischemic optic neuropathy. *Ophthalmology* 1994;101:779–782.

18 Perkin GD, Bowden P, Rose FC. Smoking and optic neuritis. *Postgrad Med* 1975;51:382–385.

19 Rizzo JF, Lessell S. Tobacco amblyopia. *Am J Ophthalmol* 1993;116:84–87.

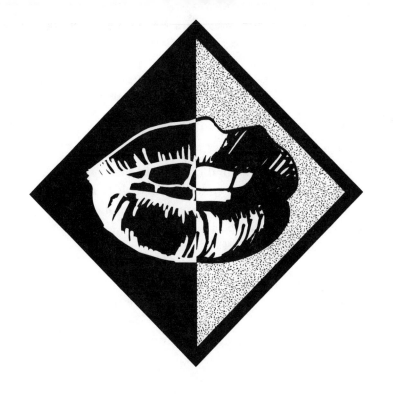

Chapter 16

SMOKING

AND ORAL HEALTH

reviewed by
Stephen J. Moss, D.D.S., M.S.
David B. Kriser Dental Center
New York, New York

Most smokers are aware that smoking causes brown teeth and bad breath. But they may be unaware that smoking-related changes in the mouth silently cause a wide range of soft tissue and periodontal diseases: diseases affecting the teeth, bone, tongue, cheeks, lips and gums.

Early studies reported that smokers had more periodontal disease simply because they had poor oral hygiene, but later studies have shown that smoking itself is a strong independent risk factor for periodontal disease.[1,2] According to some researchers, smokers have a fivefold greater risk of periodontitis[3] and are also less likely to respond to conventional treatments.[4]

How Smoking Changes the Mouth's Environment

Smoking causes a number of changes in the mouth and teeth that contribute to smokers' higher incidence of soft tissue and periodontal disease:

Smoking changes saliva: Saliva is important in maintaining the health of the oral cavity. Not only does it flush away bacteria and wastes to help keep the teeth and soft tissues healthy, but it also contains immunoglobulins, immune substances that inhibit bacterial growth and cause bacteria to clump, thus speeding their removal. The nicotine in tobacco, along with smoke's irritating and acidic nature, adversely alters saliva production.[5]

Smoking stimulates more calculus, plaque and staining: Independent of oral hygiene, smokers' teeth have a greater accumulation of plaque (soft bacterial deposits that adhere to the outer surface of the teeth)[5] and calculus (calcified deposits that form on the teeth).[2,6] Not only are these accumulations unsightly, but they act as a catchall for the subsequent collection of additional food debris and plaque.[7]

Smoking raises the temperature inside the mouth: Smoking causes the temperature inside the mouth to rise from a normal 98.6° F to 107.6° F. At this high temperature, cells are damaged and eventually die.[5]

Smoking breaks down vitamin C: This is why smokers are often found to have lower blood levels of this vitamin. In one study the average blood vitamin C level of cigarette smokers was found to be about 30 percent lower than that of nonsmokers; in those smoking more than 20 cigarettes daily, the average level was 40 percent lower.[1] This decreased vitamin C level adversely affects soft tissues within the body, impairing their ability to heal and thereby contributing to gum diseases.[1] To compensate for their habit, experts recommend that smokers need as much as 50 percent more vitamin C each day than nonsmokers.

Smoking reduces blood flow to the gingiva, or gums: The nicotine in cigarettes, once absorbed, serves as a potent peripheral vasoconstrictor. This means that blood flow to outlying parts of the body is reduced. Numerous studies have shown that smoking significantly decreases blood flow to the gums, thus preventing them from getting adequate nutrition. One study found evidence that smokers actually have fewer blood vessels in parts of their gums, which also decreases blood flow.[8] Decreased blood flow makes oral tissues more vulnerable to infection.[1,5,9,10,11]

Smoking leads to increased pocket depth. There is a space around each tooth where the gum is joined to the tooth; the depth of this space is measured as the pocket probing depth. The greater the depth, the more likely disease-causing germs are to lurk there. In addition, greater depth means there is less support to hold the tooth in place. Smokers have significantly greater pocket depths than nonsmokers.[3,10,12]

Smoking reduces response to a plaque challenge: Smokers not only have more plaque than nonsmokers, but they are also less able to respond normally to the plaque.[11] In particular, smokers fail to develop inflamed gums—gingivitis—in response to plaque accumulation as quickly as do nonsmokers.[11] Smokers thus build up more plaque on their teeth without the accompanying warning sign of inflamed, bleeding gums. The end result is that smokers have greater periodontal breakdown in response to plaque accumulation than do nonsmokers.[11]

Periodontal Diseases Associated with Smoking

Loss of alveolar bone ("tooth socket") height: Numerous studies have confirmed that smokers are more likely to lose part of the jawbone that helps hold teeth in place. This is called loss of alveolar bone height and is a well-known risk factor for tooth loss. Early tooth loss is independent of oral hygiene practices; in other words, poor oral hygiene alone does not account for smokers' greater bone loss as compared with nonsmokers.[9,13,14,15,16] Losing part of the supporting bone poses other problems, including changing the size and shape of the jaw. When this happens, the bone is less able to support dentures.

Loss of teeth: Because of one or more of the oral changes noted above, smokers are far more likely than nonsmokers to lose teeth and to have soft-tissue problems.[13,17,18]

Less success with oral surgical procedures: Smokers take longer to heal after oral surgical procedures.[5]

Acute necrotizing ulcerative gingivitis: This is a painful mouth infection indicating an overgrowth of debris and bacteria. Many adults who develop this severe form of periodontal disease are smokers.[3,5]

Cancer of the mouth, gums, lips and tongue: Smoking and other tobacco use (such as chewing) are strong predisposing factors for developing oral cancer, as described in more detail in Chapter 2.

References

1 Holmes LG. Effects of smoking and/or vitamin C on crevicular fluid flow in clinically healthy gingiva. *Quintessence International* 1990;21:191.

2 Ismail AI, Burt BA, Eklund SA. Epidemiologic patterns of smoking and periodontal disease in the United States. *JADA* 1983;106:621.

3 Stoltenberg JL, Osborn JB, Pihlstrom BL. Association between cigarette smoking, bacterial pathogens, and periodontal status. *J Periodontol* 1993;64:1225–1230.

4 Genco RJ. Assessment of risk of periodontal disease. *Compend Contin Educ Dent.* 1994; 15(suppl 18):S683.

5 Akef J. The role of smoking in the progression of periodontal disease: a literature review. *Compend Contin Educ Dent.* vol XIII (6), 528.

6 Bastiaan RJ, Waite IM. Effects of tobacco smoking on plaque development and gingivitis. *J Periodontol* 1978;49:481.

7 Peacock ME, Sutherland DE, Schuster GS. The effect of nicotine on reproduction and attachment of human gingival fibroblasts in vitro. *J Periodontol* 1993;64:658–665.

8 Danielsen B, Manji F, Nagelkerke N, et al. Effect of cigarette smoking on the transition dynamics in experimental gingivitis. *J Clin Periodontol* 1990;17:162.

9 Baab DA, Oberg PA. The effect of cigarette smoking on gingival blood flow in humans. *J Clin Periodontol* 1987; 14:418.

10 Wouters FR, et al. Significance of some variables on interproximal alveolar bone height based on cross-sectional epidemiologic data. *J Clin Periodontol* 1993;20:199–206.

11 McLaughlin WS, Lovat FM, Macgregor IDM, Kelly PJ. The immediate effects of smoking on gingival fluid flow. *J Clin Periodontol* 1993;20:448–451.

12 Locker D, Leake JL. Risk indicators and risk markers for periodontal disease experience in older adults living independently in Ontario, Canada. *J Dent Res* 1993;72:9–17.

13 Ragnarsson E, Eliasson RE, Olafsson SH. Tobacco smoking, a factor in tooth loss in Reykjavik, Iceland. *Scand J Dent Res* 1992;100:322–326.

14 Bergstrom J, Eliasson S. Cigarette smoking and alveolar bone height in subjects with a high standard of oral hygiene. *J Clin Periodontol* 1987;14:466–469.

15 Bergstrom J, Eliasson S, Preber H. Cigarette smoking and periodontal bone loss. *J Periodontol* 1991;62:242–246.

16 Ahlqwist M, Bengtsson C, Hollender L. Smoking habits and tooth loss in Swedish women. *Community Dent Oral Epidemiol* 1989;17:144–147.

17 Locker D. Smoking and oral health in older adults. *Can J Public Health* 1992;83:429.

18 Eklund SA, Burt BA. Risk factors for total tooth loss in the United States; longitudinal analysis of national data. *J Public Health Dent* 1994;54:5–14.

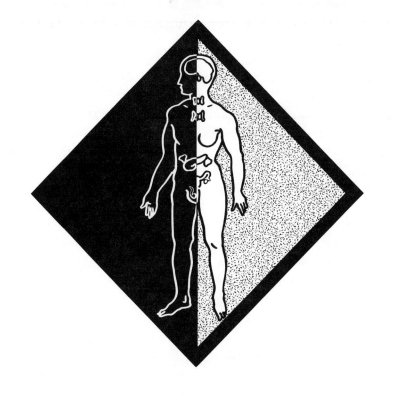

Chapter 17

SMOKING

AND THE ENDOCRINE

SYSTEM

reviewed by
Burt M. Sharp, M.D.
Professor of Medicine & Neuroscience
Departments of Medicine
Hennepin County Medical Center and University of Minnesota
Scientific Director
Institute for Brain and Immune Disorders, Minneapolis,
Minnesota

In its healthy state, the body is a finely tuned machine inside which millions of chemical reactions take place every second. Thousands of chemicals are manufactured, released and act in every cell to keep the body running and to fight disease. The endocrine system comprises the glands that are specifically designed to secrete some of these chemicals, which are called hormones. Hormones regulate distant cells and organs.

Smoking modifies the function of the endocrine system. It changes the body's metabolic rate, increases the smoker's risk of developing diabetes mellitus and even changes the way the body handles fat—a risk factor for developing heart disease and many other morbid conditions. In this chapter, we will review smoking's deleterious effects on the endocrine system.

Alterations in Body Chemical Levels

Smoking alters the body's natural release of hormones and other body chemicals. One well-known change is smoking's antiestrogenic effect; it lowers estrogen levels in a woman's body. As a result, women who smoke have an earlier menopause, which translates into an increased risk of osteoporosis and an increased risk of heart disease[1] (see Chapter 10 for a more complete description of this smoking-induced abnormality).

Levels of other body chemicals are changed by smoking as well. Catecholamines, vasopressin, endorphin and cortisol are among hormones whose levels are increased by smoking.[2] The consequences of these changes are far-reaching; they include adverse effects on blood pressure, pulse rate, metabolism and the body's reaction to physical stress.

Changed Metabolic Rate

The inverse relationship between tobacco smoking and body weight has been noted for over a century.[3] Smokers generally weigh less than nonsmokers,[4] and the ability of smoking to reduce body weight in both humans and animals is one of its most reproducible effects.[5]

Extensive studies have verified that smokers' leaner physiques are not due to their exercising more than nonsmokers; in fact, smokers are commonly less physically active than nonsmokers.[6,7] Neither are smokers' lower body weights explained by their eating less than nonsmokers; studies verify that smokers generally eat as much as or more than nonsmokers.[8,9]

Increased metabolic rate explains at least some of smokers' leaner body weights.[10] Metabolic rate is the rate at which the body burns calories and is generally expressed as calories burned per hour. Certain factors—having a fever, for example—increase the metabolic rate. Also, people who exercise regularly have higher metabolic rates than do their more sedentary counterparts.

Smoking also increases metabolic rate by approximately 2 to 10 percent; the nicotine portion is thought to be responsible.[11] And when smokers exercise, even moderately, they increase their metabolic rates even more than do nonsmokers who exercise.[9]

Experts believe that one way smoking raises metabolic rate is by stimulating the sympathetic nervous system to release more catecholamines. Among their many other effects, catecholamines cause the heart to beat faster, thus causing the body to burn more calories.[12] Nicotine also increases thermogenesis, the process by which the body produces heat. This, too, causes the body to burn more calories.[13]

But an increased metabolic rate doesn't account for the total difference in body weight between the average smoker and the average nonsmoker. Overall, smoking-induced metabolic rate increases are thought to account for about half of the difference.[14]

Another likely mechanism is that smoking alters the body-weight set point—the weight toward which a person tends to return despite vigorous attempts to gain or lose weight. This means that the changes in caloric intake that occur with changes in smoking status are actually secondary to a change in the regulation of body weight around a different set point.[15] Experts believe that smoking cessation returns the set point to normal.[9]

Abnormalities in Blood Sugar

Smoking causes abnormalities in blood sugar by at least one mechanism: Specifically, it causes a phenomenon called insulin resistance (see page 138). Insulin resistance can contribute to diabetes mellitus and to abnormalities in blood tests.

First, we'll discuss the smoker's increased risk for diabetes mellitus. Diabetes is caused both by the body's inability to produce sufficient amounts of insulin and by its inability to use effectively the insulin it has produced. Insulin is a hormone produced in the pancreas and secreted into the blood, where it serves two important functions. First, insulin increases cells' ability to use glucose, which enhances the clearance of glucose from the blood. Second, insulin inhibits the liver's production of glucose. In combination, these two functions regulate the blood sugar level.

Diabetes creates a sort of "energy crisis" in the body. Normally, glucose is "burned" as energy or is stored in the muscles and liver, in the form of glycogen, as an energy reserve. With the impaired insulin secretion or utilization that occurs in diabetes, glucose accumulates in the blood rather than being used adequately by cells as an energy source.

There are two types of diabetes. Type I, insulin-dependent diabetes mellitus (IDDM), is the more serious of the two but is also less common, accounting for just 10 percent of cases. IDDM usually strikes in childhood or adolescence and often requires multiple injections of insulin. Far more common is type II, non–insulin-dependent diabetes mellitus (NIDDM). This type generally develops in people over 40 and may be treated with diet alone; many patients may also require pills or insulin, however.

Overall, diabetes is the seventh-leading cause of death in the United States. Diabetes is associated with higher rates of cardiovascular disease, kidney disease, eye complications such as retinopathy (disorders of the retina),[16] and many other maladies.

Smoking appears to increase the risk for developing diabetes. In a recent study male smokers aged 40 to 75 were twice as likely as similarly aged nonsmokers to develop NIDDM.[16] Other researchers cite cigarette smoking as a possible independent risk factor for NIDDM in both men and women.[17]

Smokers who develop diabetes also have a markedly elevated risk of cardiovascular disease. In one study of women aged 60 to 79 who smoked and developed NIDDM, an estimated 65 percent of the cardiovascular disease deaths among the subjects were attributed to the interaction of diabetes and cigarette smoking.[18]

It is also possible that smoking precipitates fatal events in diabetics whose circulation has been compromised due to vascular disease, or blood vessels damaged by a combination of smoking and diabetes.[18]

Another phenomenon, insulin resistance, might explain the increased risk of cardiovascular disease and death among smokers who do not develop diabetes as well as among smokers who do. The cells of people who are insulin resistant cannot properly utilize insulin to burn the sugar in their blood. Extra effort, in the form of extra insulin, is needed to overcome the resistance. It's like the difference between pushing a car along a flat road and pushing it uphill.

People with insulin resistance frequently have higher than normal amounts of insulin circulating in their blood, a condition known as hyperinsulinemia. In some of these people the inability to maintain this hyperinsulinemia progresses to the development of type II diabetes. More often, though, a lack of adequate response to insulin resistance doesn't cause diabetes but results in a situation in which the body must constantly produce large amounts of insulin to *prevent* high blood sugar levels. But the body cannot do this forever. If, over time, the body produces progressively less insulin, this eventually leads to the development of diabetes.

Hyperinsulinemia may also lead to potentially dangerous abnormalities. It may raise triglycerides and lower HDL-cholesterol (the so-called "good" cholesterol), a sinister combination that significantly increases the risk for artery-clogging disease in the heart and other large blood vessels.

Several factors, genetics and obesity among them, increase a person's risk of developing insulin resistance. Smoking is also an important risk factor for insulin resistance, and risk increases with the amount smoked.[19,20] Researchers think catecholamines, which are produced in greater quantities in smokers,[21] serve as powerful antagonists to insulin action.[22] Insulin resistance is generally a chronic problem, but smoking can bring it on acutely. Smoking only six cigarettes, at a rate of two per hour, impairs insulin action in nondiabetics enough to lead to insulin resistance.[21]

Changes in the Way the Body Stores Fat

There are two distinct ways in which people carry excess body fat. So-called "apple-shaped" people carry their excess fat in the upper torso; "pear-shaped" people pack the extra pounds below the belt. Because of the location of their fat, "apples" have a higher waist-to-hip ratio (WHR) than normal. Extensive evidence has now proven that apple-shaped people have a much higher risk of developing diabetes mellitus, cardiovascular disease, hypertension, gallbladder trouble[23,24] and (in women) carcinoma of the endometrium and breast.[25]

Although smokers tend to be leaner than nonsmokers,[26] endocrine-induced changes cause smokers to store even normal amounts of body fat in an abnormal distribution, leading to an abnormally high WHR.[27,28] In one study of nearly 12,000 pre- and postmenopausal women aged 40 to 73, WHR increased as the number of cigarettes smoked per day increased.[29]

Overall, studies demonstrate a consistent dose-response relationship between number of cigarettes smoked and waist-to-hip ratio, with the ratio increasing with more cigarettes smoked. Changes in at least two hormones brought about by smoking cause this dangerous redistribution of body fat. As noted above, smoking is antiestrogenic—it causes estrogen to be destroyed faster in the liver.[30] Smoking also causes higher than normal levels of androgens to be released.[31] This smoking-affected change in sex hormones has been statistically associated with the storage of fat in the upper torso, leading to a higher WHR.[26]

References

1   Le Houezec J, Benowitz NL. Basic and clinical psychopharmacology of nicotine. *Clinics in Chest Medicine* 1991;12:681–699.

2   Wilkins JN, Carlson HE, Van Vunakis H, et al. Nicotine from cigarette smoking increases circulating levels of cortisol, growth hormone, and prolactin in male chronic smokers. *Psychopharmacology* (Berlin) 1982;78:305–308.

3   Kitchen JMW. On the value to man of the so-called divinely beneficent gift, tobacco. *Medical Record* 1889;35:459–460. As cited in Perkins KA. Effects of tobacco smoking on caloric intake. *Br J Addiction* 1992;87:193–205.

4   Albanes D, Jones Y, Micozzi M, Mattson M. Associations between smoking and body weight in the US population. *Am J Public Health* 1987;77:439–444.

5   Grunberg NW, Bowen DJ, Maycock VA, Nespor SM. The importance of sweet taste and caloric content in the effects of nicotine on specific food consumption. *Psychopharmacology* 1985;87:198–203.

6   Blair S, Jacobs D, Powell KE. Relationships between exercise or physical activity and other health behaviors. *Public Health Rep* 1985;100:172–180.

7   Marks BL, Perkins KA, Metz KF, et al. Effects of smoking status on content of caloric intake and energy expenditure. *International Journal on Eating Disorders* 1991;10:441–449.

8   Hughes JR, Higgins ST, Hatsukami D. Effects of abstinence from tobacco. In: Kozlowski LT, et al., eds. *Research Advances in Alcohol and Drug Problems* 1990;10:317–398.

9   Perkins KA. Weight gain following smoking cessation. *J Consulting Clin Psychol* 1993;61:768–777.

10 Dallosso HM, James WPT. The role of smoking in the regulation of energy balance. *International Journal of Obesity* 1984;8:365–375.

11 Perkins KA. Metabolic effects of cigarette smoking. *J Applied Psychol* 1992b;72:401–409.

12 Jarvik ME. Beneficial effects of nicotine. *Br J Addiction* 1991;86:571–575.

13 Yoshida T, Yoshioka K, Kiraoka N, Kondo M. Effect of nicotine on norepinephrine turnover and thermogenesis in brown adipose tissue and metabolic rate in MSG obese mice. *J Nutritional Sci Vitaminol* 1990;36:123–130.

14 Hofstetter A, Schutz Y, Jequier E, Wahren J. Increased 24-hour energy expenditure in cigarette smokers. *N Engl J Med* 1986;314:79–82.

15 Perkins KA, Denier CA, Mayer JA, Scott RR, Dubbert PM. Weight gain associated with reductions in smoking rate and nicotine content. *International Journal of Addictions* 1987a;22:578–581.

16 Rimm EB, Chan J, Stampfer MJ, et al. Prospective study of cigarette smoking, alcohol use, and the risk of diabetes in men. *Br Med J* 1995;310:555.

17 Feskens EJM, Kromhout D. Cardiovascular risk factors and the 25-year incidence of diabetes mellitus in middle-age men: the Zutphen study. *Am J Epidemiol* 1989;130:1101–1108. Also, Rimm EB, Manson JE, Stampfer MJ, et al. Cigarette smoking and the risk of diabetes in women. *Am J Public Health* 1993;83:211–214. Both as cited in Eliasson B, Attvall S, et al. The insulin resistance syndrome in smokers is related to smoking habits. *Arteriosclerosis and Thrombosis* 1994;14;1946–1950.

18 Suarez L, Barrett-Connor E. Interaction between cigarette smoking and diabetes mellitus in the prediction of death attributed to cardiovascular disease. *Am J Epidemiol* 1984;120:670–675.

19 Eliasson B, Attvall S, Taskinen M-R, Smith U. The insulin resistance syndrome in smokers is related to smoking habits. *Arteriosclerosis and Thrombosis* 1994;14:1946–1950.

20 Attvall S, Fowelin J, Lager I, von Schenck H, Smith U. Smoking induces insulin resistance: a potential link with the insulin resistance syndrome. *J Intern Med* 1993;233:327–332.

21 Cryer PE, Haymond MW, Santiago JV, Shah SD. Norepinephrine and epinephrine release and andrengergic mediation of smoking-associated hemodynamic and metabolic events. *N Engl J Med* 1976;295: 573–577.

22 Lager I, Attvall S, Eriksson BM, von Schenk H, Smith U. Studies of the insulin-antagonistic effect of catecholamines in normal man: evidence for the importance of beta receptors. *Diabetologia* 1986;29:409–416.

23 Folsom AR, Kaye SA, Sellers TA, et al. Body fat distribution and 5-year risk of death in older women. *JAMA* 1993;269:483–487.

24 van der Kooy K, Leenen R, Seidell JC, et al. Waist-hip ratio is a poor predictor of changes in visceral fat. *Am J Clin Nutr* 1993;57:327–333.

25 Kaye SA, Folsom AR, Prineas RJ, Potter JD, Gapstur SD. The association of body fat distribution with lifestyle and reproductive factors in a population study of postmenopausal women. *International Journal of Obesity* 1990;14:583–591.

26 Lew EA, Garfinkel L. Variations in mortality by weight among 750,000 men and women. *J Chron Dis* 1979;32:563–576.

27 Gossain VV, Sherma NK, Srivastava L, et al. Hormonal effects of smoking II: effects on plasma cortisol, growth hormone and prolactin. *Am J Med Sci* 1986;291:325–327.

28 Armellini F, Zamboni M, Frigo L, Mandragona R, Robbi R, Micciolo R, Bosello O. Alcohol consumption, smoking habits and body fat distribution in Italian men and women aged 20–60 years. *European Journal of Clinical Nutrition* 1993;47:52–60.

29 den Tonkelaar I, Seidell JC, van Noord P, Baanders-van Halewijn EA, Ouwehand IJ. Fat distribution in relation to age, degree of obesity, smoking habits, parity and estrogen use: a cross-sectional study in 11,825 Dutch women participating the DOM project. *International Journal of Obesity* 1990;14:753–761.

30 Baer L, Radickerich I. Cigarette smoking in hypertensive patients—blood pressure and endocrine response. *Am J Med* 1985;78:564–568. As cited in den Tonkelaar, et al. Fat distribution in relation to age, degree of obesity, smoking habits, parity and estrogen use. *International Journal of Obesity* 1990;14:753–761.

31 Khaw K, Tazuda S, Barrett-Connor E. Cigarette smoking and levels of adrenal androgens in postmenopausal women. *N Engl J Med* 1988;318:1705–1708.

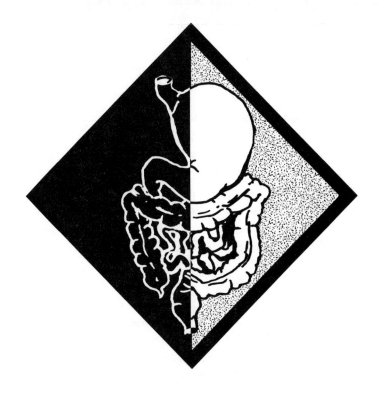

Chapter 18

SMOKING

AND GASTROINTESTINAL

DISEASES

reviewed by
Steven D. Wexner, M.D.
Chairman, Department of Colorectal Surgery
Cleveland Clinic Florida

Smoking exerts powerful effects on the gastrointestinal system: It causes the stomach to produce more acid, changes its ability to fight disease-causing organisms and alters blood flow to tissues. Smoking also stimulates changes in the intestine that lead to a greater risk of several diseases. Ultimately, smoking influences disease risk from the mouth (it increases the risk of cancer) to the stomach (it raises ulcer and cancer risk) all the way through the GI tract to the rectum (it increases the risk of colon polyps, cancer and the inflammatory bowel condition known as Crohn's disease).

In this chapter we will review the multiple and serious noncancerous effects of smoking on the gastrointestinal tract. (We discussed the role smoking plays in causing cancer of the colon—the second leading cause of cancer death in the United States—in Chapter 2.)

How Smoking Affects the Tissues of the Gastrointestinal Tract

Smoking Increases the Risk of Stomach Ulcers

Smoking has long been linked with an increased risk of stomach, or peptic, ulcers; with greater difficulty in treating the ulcers; and with a higher chance of ulcer recurrence. While both heavy and light smokers have more peptic ulcer disease, risk accelerates with increasing pack-years of cigarette smoking.[1,2]

In one study the smoking-related excess risk for peptic ulcer was statistically significant in all age groups. In that study 25.4 percent—one quarter—of the peptic ulcers diagnosed for the first time in people aged 35 to 84 were estimated to be caused by smoking, as were 42 percent—nearly half—of relapsing ulcers.[3] Other researchers have estimated that 20 percent of all peptic ulcer cases among U.S. women are attributable to cigarette smoking.[2]

Smoking raises ulcer risk by several mechanisms. It causes the stomach to produce more acid and pepsin (a digestive enzyme),[4] but most researchers say that this increased acid and pepsin production doesn't entirely explain smokers' increased incidence of stomach ulcers. While daytime stomach-acid production is indeed higher in smokers than in nonsmokers, there is often no difference in nighttime acidity between the two groups. The difference in stomach acidity between smokers and nonsmokers occurs for just part of the day and is thus too small to explain the entire phenomenon.[5]

But there are other changes caused by smoking that increase ulcer risk. These changes work in conjunction with the slightly increased acidity. Among the other contributing factors are these:

- The nicotine in tobacco smoke, in addition to increasing acid production, impairs the stomach's ability to neutralize acid after a meal. While stomach acid is vital to food breakdown and digestion, the healthy body has an amazing ability to neutralize the acid after food is digested. This neutralization protects the lining of the stomach from damage that could occur because of prolonged acid exposure. In smokers, however, neutralization is impaired. As a result, stomach acidity stays higher for longer periods and contributes to ulcer risk by "eating away" at the stomach lining.[6]

- Chronic nicotine intake also wreaks havoc with blood circulation in the stomach lining; doctors refer to this as dysregulation of the gastric microcirculation. This impaired blood circulation in turn causes biochemical changes in the tissues of the stomach, weakening them and making them more prone to damage by even slightly increased acid production. And impaired blood flow not only increases ulcer risk; it is also a factor in delayed ulcer healing.[7]

- The extremely high nicotine concentrations in the gastric juices of smokers alter the cytoprotective properties of the mucosa (the mucous membrane). This means that smoking decreases immunity, lowering resistance to infection.[8] As a result, smokers are more prone to becoming infected with a bacterium, *Helicobacter pylori,* that is associated with an increased risk of developing ulcers.[9] In smokers and nonsmokers alike, clearing up an *H. pylori* infection helps cure the ulcer.

- Smoking may also have a direct toxic effect on epithelial cells, the cells lining the stomach. Because this toxic effect causes the stomach lining to become weakened, it may be more susceptible to damage by stomach acid.

- Cigarette smokers have significantly more gastric reflux than do nonsmokers. The acid from a smoker's stomach backs up, creating the sense of heartburn. This in turn increases the chance of the smoker's getting an ulcer; it also lowers the ulcer healing rate. Gastric reflux is, in fact, present much more often in smokers than in nonsmokers— even when the smokers are not actually smoking.[10]

- Older people who smoke produce significantly less of a naturally occurring substance called gastric prostaglandin. Among other things, prostaglandins protect tissues from damage. Because these older smokers produce less gastric prostaglandin, they have yet another risk factor for stomach ulcers.[11] (Prostaglandin production is also reduced in the duodenum of smokers; see below.)

Smoking Increases the Risk of Duodenal Ulcers

Smoking is associated with an increased risk of duodenal ulcer, an ulcer in the portion of the small intestine that connects to the stomach. As with stomach ulcers, duodenal ulcers in smokers increase with the number of pack-years of cigarette smoking,[1] have a high relapse rate and are difficult to treat. Even ex-smokers are at increased risk for slow healing of duodenal ulcers.[12]

As in the case of stomach ulcers, factors other than increased acid and pepsin production are responsible for smokers' increased risk of duodenal ulcers. The other factors that play a role are as follows:

- There is greater incidence in smokers of both *Helicobacter pylori* infections and nicotine-induced damage to the epithelial cells that line the duodenum; both are thought to play a role in the increased risk of duodenal ulcers noted in smokers.[8]

- Cigarette smoking markedly inhibits the secretion of bicarbonate, a substance that helps neutralize stomach acid.[13]

- Smoking reduces the amount of prostaglandin produced in the duodenum, creating yet another risk factor for duodenal ulcer.[14]

While medications are often less effective and are required in higher doses to treat both stomach and duodenal ulcers in smokers,[15] much of the research on this subject has been done on how those medications respond in smokers with duodenal ulcers. In summary:

- To have complete healing and to prevent relapse, smokers with duodenal ulcers generally need double the dose required by nonsmokers of a medication called rantidine (Zantac).[16]

- Two other medications used for duodenal ulcers, cimetidine (Tagamet) and Mylanta II, do not work as well in smokers.[17]

- Duodenal ulcer patients who are smokers and who receive cimetidine do not heal well unless they also receive a medication called sucralfate (Carafate); this combined medication regimen is generally not necessary in nonsmokers.[18]

- Similarly, nizatidine, another drug used to promote healing and prevent relapse in duodenal ulcers, does not work as well in smokers.[19]

Smoking Increases the Risk of Crohn's Disease

Smoking increases the risk of developing the chronic inflammatory bowel condition called Crohn's disease.[20] People who have this disease suffer bouts of severe diarrhea and intestinal bleeding, problems that can originate in the small and/or the large intestine. The disease often becomes so severe that sufferers must have part of their intestine removed; some people go through multiple surgeries. Smokers not only have a greater risk of developing the disease; they also have a greater risk of suffering much worse disease.

The risk of Crohn's disease increases with the number of packs smoked per day.[20] In one study women who were current smokers had a fivefold increased risk of Crohn's disease.[21] The use of chewing tobacco also increases the risk of developing Crohn's disease by at least twofold. People who both use snuff and smoke cigarettes have an estimated 3.7-fold increased risk over people who neither chew nor smoke.[22]

Continued smoking after a diagnosis of Crohn's disease increases the likelihood of the smoker's suffering a first relapse[23] as well as a recurrence at any time.[24] Continued smoking also significantly worsens the course of the disease.[25] Crohn's patients who smoke suffer more serious complications and report significantly more days on which their illness troubles them over the course of a month than do nonsmokers. In one study smokers reported 15.4 troubled days per month versus five troubled days for nonsmokers.[26]

While many patients with Crohn's disease need surgery because of complications of their disease, patients who smoke more than 10 cigarettes per day are more likely to need both a first and subsequent surgery because of serious complications. The risk of needing surgery continues to grow with persistent smoking. If smoking continues for more than 10 years, the risk of the smoker's needing more than one surgery is nearly doubled as compared with the risk in a nonsmoker. In addition, Crohn's patients who continue to smoke have a greatly increased chance of suffering an abscess, a serious bowel infection.[25]

Smoking Increases the Risk of Colon Polyps
Smokers also increase their risk of developing growths called polyps in their colons. In one study there was an association between smoking and polyps of a certain size but not of other sizes. In particular, the risk was greatest for polyps larger than one centimeter in diameter.[27] Because some colon polyps go on to become cancerous, this association between polyps and smoking is important.

Smoking Decreases but Chewing Increases the Risk of Ulcerative Colitis
Ulcerative colitis is a chronic condition that causes diarrhea and bleeding in the large intestine. The literature clearly indicates that cigarette smoking actually protects against this inflammatory bowel condition (see below); but the use of chewing tobacco, either alone or with smoking, increases the risk of developing the disease. Compared with those who don't use chewing tobacco, chewers face a doubled risk of developing ulcerative colitis. The risk jumps to 3.3 for people who use chewing tobacco and also smoke as compared with those who use neither product.[22]

Protection Against Disease
While nicotine causes many serious and often fatal illnesses throughout the body, it offers protection against some diseases. In the gastrointestinal

tract it provides protection against ulcerative colitis, but only in smokers who don't also use chewing tobacco.[28]

Compared with lifetime nonsmokers, smokers have a reduced risk of ulcerative colitis. Ulcerative colitis is, in fact, largely a disease of non-smokers. Curiously, the risk is increased in ex-smokers. People who stop smoking have a four- to eightfold increased risk of developing ulcerative colitis as compared with people who have never smoked.[29,30]

Anecdotal evidence suggests that nicotine may alleviate symptoms of ulcerative colitis. Researchers have found that the use of transdermal nicotine patches in conjunction with conventional therapy improves symptoms of the disease. Experts think the nicotine works on the symptoms by changing the inflammatory process or by altering the mucus membranes in the colon and rectum.[31,32] Alternatively, because nicotine reduces blood flow to the colon and rectum, it may reduce the inflammatory substances that reach the mucous membranes of the tissues there.[33]

References

1 Kato I, Nomura AMY, Stemmermann GN, Chyou PH. A prospective study of gastric and duodenal ulcer and its relation to smoking, alcohol and diet. *Am J Epidemiol* 1992;135:521–530.

2 Anda R, Williamson D, Escobedo L, Remington P. Smoking and the risk of peptic ulcer disease among women in the United States. *Arch Intern Med* 1990;150:1437–1441.

3 Schoon I, Mellstrom D, Oden A, Ytterberg B. Peptic ulcer disease in older age groups in Gothenburg in 1985: the association with smoking. *Age and Aging* 1991;20:371–376.

4 Lanas A, Hirschowitz BI. Influence of smoking on basal and vagally and maximally stimulated gastric acid and pepsin secretion. *Scand J Gastroenterol* 1992;27:208–212.

5 Kaufmann D, Wilder–Smith CH, Kempf M, Neumann J, Schmolls H, Witzel L, Walt RP, Rohmel J, Merki HS. Cigarette smoking, gastric acidity and peptic ulceration: what are the relationships? *Dig Dis Sci* 1990;35:1482–1487.

6 Lindell G, Brudin L, Ohlin P, Graffner H. Does nicotine administration influence intragastric acidity? *Scand J Gastroenterol* 1992;27:143–146.

7 Battistel M, Plebani M, Di Mario F, Jocic M, Lippe IT, Holzer P. Chronic nicotine intake causes vascular dysregulation in the rat gastric mucosa. *Gut* 1993;34:1688–1692.

8 Lindell G, Farnebo O, Chen D, Nexo E, Madsen J, Bukhave K, Graffner H. Acute effects of smoking during modified sham feeding in duodenal ulcer patients. *Scand J Gastroenterol* 1993;28:487–494.

9 Bateson, M C. Cigarette smoking and Heliocobacter pylori infection. *Postgraduate Medical Journal* 1993;69:41–44.

10 Muller-Lissner S. Bile reflux is increased in cigarette smokers. *Gastroenterology* 1986;90:1205–1209.

11 Cryer B, Lee E, Feldman M. Factors influencing gastroduodenal mucosal prostaglandin concentrations: roles of smoking and aging. *Ann Intern Med* 1992;116:636–640.

12 Armstrong D, Arnold R, Classen M, Fischer M, Goebell H, Blum A. The Ruder Study Group. Prospective multicentre study of risk factors associated with delayed healing of recurrent duodenal ulcers (RUDER). *Gut* 1993;34:1319–1326.

13 Ainsworth M, Hogan D, Koss M, Isenberg J. Cigarette smoking inhibits acid-stimulated duodenal mucosal bicarbonate secretion. *Ann Intern Med* 1993;119:882–886.

14 Cryer B, Lee E, Feldman M. Factors influencing gastroduodenal mucosal prostaglandin concentrations: roles of smoking and aging. *Ann Intern Med* 1992;116:636–640.

15 Korman M, Hansky J, Merrett A, et al. Ranitidine in duodenal ulcer: influence of healing and effect on smoking. *Dig Dis Sci* 1982;27:712–715.

16 Lee F, Hardman M, Jaderberg M. Maintenance treatment of duodenal ulceration: ranitidine 300 mg at night is better than 150 mg in cigarette smokers. *Gut* 1991;32:151–153.

17 Korman M, Shaw R, Hansky J, et al. Influence of smoking on the healing rate of duodenal ulcer in response to cimetidine or high-dose antacid. *Gastroenterology* 1981;80:1451–1453.

18 Lam SK, Hui WM, Lau WY, et al. Sucralfate overcomes adverse effect of cigarette smoking on duodenal ulcer healing and prolongs subsequent remission. *Gastroenterology* 1987;92:1193–1201.

19 Kuipers E, Hazenberg H, Quik R, et al. Nizatidine versus ranitidine in the treatment of peptic ulcer disease: report on the Dutch investigation as part of a European multicentre trial. *Netherlands J Med* 1990;37:58–62.

20 Lashner BA, Shaheen NJ, Hanauer SB, Kirschner BS. Passive smoking is associated with an increased risk of developing inflammatory bowel disease in children. *Am J Gastroenterol* 1993;88:356–359.

21 Tragnone A, Hanau C, Bazzochi G, et al. Epidemiological characteristics of inflammatory bowel disease in Bologna, Italy—incidence and risk factors. *Digestion* 1993;54:183–188.

22 Persson PG, Hellers G, Ahlbom A. Use of oral moist snuff and inflammatory bowel disease. *Int J Epidemiol* 1993;22:1101–1103.

23 Wright JP. Factors influencing first relapse in patients with Crohn's disease. *J Clin Gastroenterol* 1992;15:12–16.

24 Cottone M, Rosselli M, Orlando A, et al. Smoking habits and recurrence in Crohn's disease. *Gastroenterology* 1994;106:643–648.

25 Lindberg E, Jarnerot G, Huitfeldt B. Smoking in Crohn's disease: effect on localisation and clinical course. *Gut* 1992;33:779–782.

26 Kurata JH, Kantor-Fish S, Frankl H, et al. Crohn's disease among ethnic groups in a large health maintenance organization. *Gastroenterology* 1992;102:1940–1948.

27 Zahm S, Cocco P, Blair A. Tobacco smoking as a risk factor for colon polyps. *Am J Public Health* 1991;81:846–849.

28 Jarvik M. Beneficial effects of nicotine. *Br J Addiction* 1991;86:571–575.

29 Tysk C, Jarnerot G. Has smoking changed the epidemiology of ulcerative colitis? *Scand J Gastroenterol* 1992;27:508–512.

30 Samuelsson S, Ekbom A, Zack M, Helmick C, Adami H. Risk factors for extensive ulcerative colitis and ulcerative proctitis: a population based case–control study. *Gut* 1991;32:1526–1530.

31 Pullan R, Rhodes J, Ganesh S, et al. Transdermal nicotine for active ulcerative colitis. *N Engl J Med* 1994;330:811–815.

32 Zijlstra F, Srivastava E, Rhodes M, et. al. Effect of nicotine on rectal mucus and mucosal eicosanoids. *Gut* 1994;35:247–251.

33 Srivastava E, Russell M, Feyerabend C, Rhodes J. Effects of ulcerative colitis and smoking on rectal blood flow. *Gut* 1990;31:1021–1024.

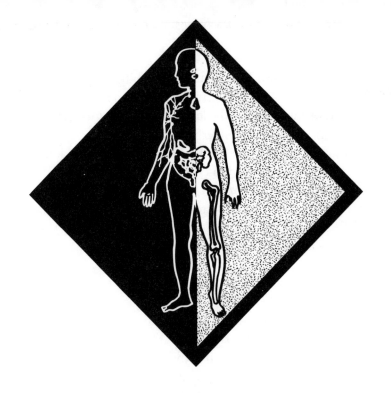

Chapter 19

SMOKING

AND THE IMMUNE

SYSTEM

reviewed by
Arnold Levinson, M.D.
University of Pennsylvania
Philadelphia, Pennsylvania

Smoking impairs the immune system—the body's critical defense against such invading organisms as infectious agents and allergy-provoking substances. As a result, smokers suffer more infections, including respiratory infections and infections after surgery, than do nonsmokers. Smoking even impairs immunity in the mouth, leading to more periodontal disease. Smokers also suffer more (and more serious) allergic reactions.

In this chapter we will review the evidence of smoking's negative effects on the human immune system and, when the mechanisms have been identified, explain why. First, though, we begin with a brief description of the normal human immune system.

The Normal Immune System

The immune system is divided into two main parts, the humoral immune system and the cellular immune system.

The humoral component fights infection through a system of antibodies that work to combat antigens. Antigens are foreign substances such as bacteria, viruses and allergy-producing substances (pollen, for example). The humoral system produces antibodies in response to an invasion by antigens. Each of the several types of antibodies is a specific type of immunoglobulin. There are five main categories of immunoglobulins in humans: IgA, IgD, IgE, IgG and IgM. Each is made up of a specific sequence of amino acids in the region that binds the antigen. This unique pattern enables each immunoglobulin to bind the specific antigen that stimulates its production. Some antibodies fight infections by binding and disabling infection-causing antigens. Others induce the allergy response when they bind pollen and other allergy-inducing antigens.

The other system is the cellular immune system, also called cell-mediated immunity. This aggregate works through cells known as T cells or T lymphocytes, which are lymphocytes produced in the thymus gland. There are many types of T cells vital to cellular immunity; they include memory, helper, suppressor and killer cells. Each type of T cell plays an important, specific and irreplaceable role in the normal immune response, which means that maintaining the proper distribution of T cells is critical to mounting a normal immune response.

The humoral and cellular immune systems work together in a complex relationship, policing the body for foreign substances and keeping it healthy. But there also are many other cells that are important in the scheme of immunity. Among these are other leukocytes, or white blood cells, that lack specificity of action. These cells are found in the blood at various stages of development, and cells at each of these stages function in different capacities to fight infections and other foreign substances. Included in this category are neutrophils, eosinophils and monocytes. Cells known as macrophages are also important in immunity; among other things, they phagocytize, or "gobble up," antigens.

How Smoking Changes the Immune System

Smoking causes many changes in the body's complex immune system. And while just one change is enough to impair the immune system, several can be disastrous. Either alone or together, these changes and impairments place smokers at a higher risk of infections and allergies.

The changes caused by smoking can be divided into four categories: those that impair the humoral immune system, those that impair cell-mediated immunity, those that have negative effects on the nonspecific leukocytes and those that impair other cells of the immune system.

Impairments to Humoral Immunity
Smoking's impairments to humoral immunity include:

- Increased levels of IgE in the blood. Because this particular antibody plays an important role in allergic reactions, an increase in IgE might place smokers at increased risk of suffering allergic reactions. Also, smokers do not exhibit the seasonal changes in IgE levels that nonsmokers do. (In nonsmokers, IgE levels are lower in the winter and summer, when there is less pollen in the air). Immunologists think the overabundance of IgE in smokers' blood might be due to the fact that smoking suppresses the number and normal functioning of one category of T lymphocytes, the regulatory T lymphocytes. Among other important jobs, the regulatory T cells help control the amounts of immunoglobulins produced.[1]

- Decreased blood levels of the immunoglobulins IgA, IgG and IgM.[2,3] Of all the places in the body in which immunoglobulins exist, a lack in the blood is the most serious; it predisposes the smoker to more infections. Too little IgG, for example, can predispose a smoker to more respiratory infections.

- Decreased concentration of antibodies in nasal mucosa (the mucous membrane). This decreased concentration means that smokers are deficient in their first line of defense against respiratory germs.[4] This corresponds with the finding that smokers show an impaired response to antigens encountered by nasal and respiratory mucosa.[5]

- Decreased amounts of IgA and IgG in saliva.[6] This decreases a smoker's ability to destroy germs that enter through the mouth.

Impairments to Cell-Mediated Immunity
These include:

- An increased number of T lymphocytes, but in an abnormal distribution. While the total number of T cells is increased in smokers,[1] the distribution of the subsets of T cells is altered. In particular, there are fewer T helper-inducer cells, and more T suppressor-cytotoxic cells.[7] As noted previously, maintaining the optimal distribution of T-cell subtypes is essential to mounting a strong immune defense.

- An increased number of chromosomally injured lymphocytes in the blood.[8] Because chromosomes contain the genetic information necessary to reproduce normally, cells that are not chromosomally normal have a greater chance of reproducing damaged copies.

- Inhibited proliferation of T lymphocytes. This ability to proliferate is essential to maintaining a normally functioning immune system. Smoking, however, inhibits lymphocyte proliferation.[9]

Negative Effects on Nonspecific Leukocytes
These include:

- An increased number of total white blood cells. Smokers have about

30 percent more white blood cells than nonsmokers. This may reflect the greater number of infections they suffer.[1]

• Fewer natural killer cells.[6] Natural killer cells play an important part in checking the growth of tumor cells and cells infected with some viruses. They play a more significant role in regulating the growth of cells from which white cells originate.

• Impaired neutrophil function. It is thought that smoking exerts direct toxic effects on neutrophils, another type of leukocytes. Among its most important effects, cigarette smoke impairs the neutrophils' ability to move properly. It also impairs their metabolic machinery—their inner workings. The most significant impact of impaired neutrophil function in smokers is an increased rate of respiratory infections.[10]

• Impaired polymorphonuclear lymphocytes (PMNs) in the bloodstream. Smoking impairs the ability of PMNs to migrate, or move, normally[10] and also impairs their ability to phagocytize (consume) antigens.[11]

• Disabled PMNs in gum tissue. PMNs are the first line of defense in inflammatory responses in the gums or gingival tissue, such as occur with gum or periodontal disease. The mouth is dependent on these cells to phagocytize plaque.[12] Lacking normally functioning PMNs, the smoker is more likely to suffer periodontal disease.

• An increased number of eosinophils. This abnormality has several consequences, including impaired lung functioning (especially in the lower lung tissue), increased respiratory symptoms and a worsening of the symptoms of smokers who have emphysema (a chronic, progressive lung condition that makes it difficult for the sufferer to get enough oxygen into the lungs). An increase in the number of eosinophils is associated with allergy-induced inflammation.[1]

Impairments to Other Cells of the Immune System
Smoking changes the shape, metabolic activity and functioning of macrophages,[13] rendering them far less capable of consuming antigens.

How These Changes Affect the Risk of Disease
As well as increasing the risk of bronchitis, pneumonia and other respiratory-tract infections, the changes to the components of the immune system that are brought about by smoking result in an increased risk for other diseases. Among these other consequences are the following:

- an increased risk of acquiring epidemic influenza[14,15];

- a decreased response to hepatitis B vaccine (which means the vaccine isn't as effective)[16];

- an apparent increased risk of varicella pneumonia, a type of pneumonia that results from chicken pox[17];

- a less effective response to influenza or flu vaccination (which means that the flu vaccine doesn't work as well in smokers).[1]

Smoking and AIDS
While some studies suggest that smoking causes HIV-1–infected people to progress more quickly to AIDS (a disease characterized by severe immune system dysfunction), the results have not been consistent. Of the seven identified studies, two indicated that smoking does cause an earlier progression to AIDS,[18,19] four failed to find an association[20,21,22,23] and one found that smoking alters immune function but doesn't change the clinical course of the disease.[24]

References

1   Sherman C. The health consequences of cigarette smoking: pulmonary diseases. *Med Clin North Am* 1992;76:355–375.

2   Gerrard JW, Heiner DC, Mink J, et al. Immunoglobulin levels in smokers and non-smokers. *Ann Allergy* 1980;44:261–262.

3   Srivastava ED, Barton JR, O'Mahony S, et al. Smoking, humoral immunity and ulcerative colitis. *Gut* 1991;32:1016–1019.

4   Rylander R, Wold A, Haglind P. Nasal antibodies against Gram-negative bacteria in cotton-mill workers. *Int Arch Allergy Appl Immunol* 1982;69:330–333.

5   Anderson P, Pederson OF, Bach B, Bonde GJ. Serum antibodies and immunoglobulins in smokers and nonsmokers. *Clin Exp Immunol* 1982;47:467–473.

6   Ferson M, Edwards A, Lind A, et al. Low natural killer-cell activity and immunoglobulin levels associated with smoking in human subjects. *Int J Cancer* 1979;23:603–609.

7   Miller LG, Goldstein G, Murphy M, Ginns LC. Reversible alterations in immunoregulatory T-cells in smoking. *Crest* 1982;82:526–529.

8   Tucker JD, Ashworth IK, Johnston GR, et al. Variation in the human lymphocyte sister chromatid exchange frequency: results of a long term longitudinal study. *Mutation Research* 1988;204:435–444.

9   Desplaces A, Charreire J, Izard C; as cited in Corberand J, Nguyen F, Do AH, et al. Effect of tobacco smoking on the functions of polymorphonuclear leukocytes. *Infection and Immunity* 1979;23:577–581.

10 Corberand J, Nguyen F, Do AH, et al. Effect of tobacco smoking on the functions of polymorphonuclear leukocytes. *Infection and Immunity* 1979;23:577–581.

11 Kenney EB, Karaal JK, Saxe SR, Jones J. The effect of cigarette smoking on human oral polymorphonuclear leukocytes. *J Periodontal Research* 1977;12:227–234.

12 Akef J, Weine FS, Weissman DP. The role of smoking in the progression of periodontal disease: a literature review. *Compend Contin Educ Dent.* vol XIII, no. 6:526–530.

13 Chretien J, Thieblemont M, Masse R, et al. as cited in Corberand J, Nguyen F, Do AH, et al. *Infection and Immunity* 1979;23:577–581.

14 Finklea JF, Sandifer SH, Smith DD. Cigarette smoking and epidemic influenza. *Am J Epidemiol* 1969;90:390–399.

15 Finklea JF, Hasselblad V, Riggan WB, et al. Cigarette smoking and hemagglutination inhibition response to influenza after natural disease and immunization. *Am Rev Resp Dis* 1971;104:368–376.

16 Horowitz MM, Ershler WB, McKinney WP, et al. Duration of immunity after hepatitis B vaccination: efficacy of low dose booster vaccine. *Ann Intern Med* 1988;108:185–189.

17 Ellis ME, Neal KR, Webb AK. Is smoking a risk factor for pneumonia in adults with chickenpox? *Br Med J* 1987;294:1002 (letter).

18 Nieman RB, Fleming J, Coker RJ, et al. The effect of cigarette smoking on the development of AIDS in HIV-1 seropositive individuals. *AIDS* 1993;7:705–710.

19 Royce R, Winkelstein W Jr. HIV infection, cigarette smoking and CD4+ T-lymphocyte counts: preliminary results from the San Francisco Men's Health Study. *AIDS* 1990;4:327–333.

20 Park LP, Margolick JB, Giorgi JV, et al. Influence of HIV-1 infection and cigarette smoking on leukocyte profiles in homosexual men. The Multicenter AIDS Cohort Study. *J Acquir Immune Defic Syndr* 1992;5:1124–1130.

21 Craib KJ, Schecter MT, Le TN, et al. Effect of cigarette smoking on CD4 count and progression to AIDS in a cohort of homosexual men. VII International Conference on AIDS. Florence, 1991;MC 3110.

22 Eskild A, Petersen G. Cigarette smoking and drinking of alcohol are not associated with rapid progression to acquired immunodeficiency syndrome among homosexual men in Norway. *Scand J Soc Med* 1994;22:209–212.

23 Coberly J, Cantave M, Quinn T, et al. The effects of age, sex and smoking on temporal changes in CD4 and beta-2-microglobulin levels in HIV seropositive and seronegative Haitian adults. Int Conf AIDS. 1992 July 19–24;8(2):C308 (abstract no. PoC 4383).

24 Burns DN, Dramer A, Yellin F, et al. Cigarette smoking: a modifier of human immunodeficiency virus type I infection. *J Acquir Immune Defic Syndr* 1991;4:76–83.

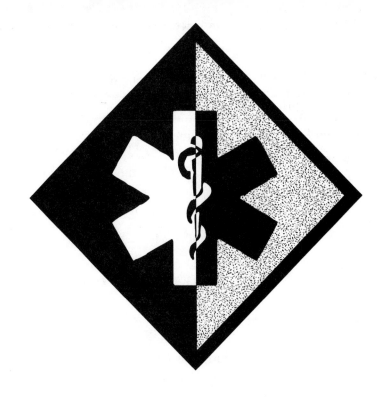

Chapter 20

SMOKING

AND EMERGENCY

MEDICINE

reviewed by
Stephen K. Epstein, M.D., M.P.P.
Associate in Medicine, Harvard Medical School
Attending Physician, Division of Emergency Medicine
Beth Israel Hospital, Boston,
Massachusetts

In addition to the long-term consequences of smoking discussed in the previous chapters, there can be other, immediate, negative health consequences of smoking. The most devastating of these are the injuries and deaths related to fires started by smoking materials. In this chapter we will also discuss other, non–fire-related, injuries associated with smoking; these include injuries incurred in auto crashes and those incurred in smokers' occupational settings. We are including them in the emergency medicine chapter because all injuries—whether caused by a fire, an auto crash or a work-related accident—are treated by emergency-medicine personnel.

Smoking-Associated Fires

Smoking materials (especially cigarettes) are the leading cause of fire deaths in the United States and are responsible for 28 percent of all household fire deaths.[1] Put another way, more than one of every four fire deaths in the United States can be attributed to smoking materials.

According to the National Fire Protection Association,[1] 163,100 fires were caused by cigarettes and other smoking-material fires in 1992, the latest year for which figures are available. As a result of these fires, 1,075 people died and 3,232 were injured.

In addition to being the leading cause of fire deaths, smoking is the second-leading cause of injuries related to household fires, ranking second only to injuries caused by cooking-equipment fires. In 1992 the loss in property from these fires totaled $318 million.[2]

Smoking and Car Accidents

Research reveals that people who smoke are more likely to be involved in car crashes for which they are responsible. Interestingly, while this risk certainly is increased for those who smoke while they are driving, it is also elevated among smokers who are not smoking at the time of their crash (researchers have not discerned exactly why). According to one case-control study, smokers had a 1.5-fold increased risk for at-fault crashes.[3] Whether this increased accident risk is due to the pharmacological effects of nicotine and other chemicals in cigarettes, to being distracted by lighting or handling the cigarette, or to some combination of the two, has not been defined.[4]

Smoking and Other Injuries

Occupational injuries. According to the National Center for Injury Prevention and Control, smokers, in addition to being more likely to be involved in car accidents, are also 1.4 to 2.5 times more likely to be injured at work.[5]

As reviewed by researchers Sacks and Nelson,[5] a study of employees at one petrochemical company demonstrated that smokers had 2.5 times the incidence of occupational injuries as nonsmokers. In another study cited by Sacks and Nelson, postal employees who smoked had a 1.4 times increased risk for occupational injuries even after controlling for age, sex, race, drug use, job classification and exercise.

Other Unintentional Injuries. Also as reviewed by Sacks and Nelson,[5] smokers are more likely than nonsmokers to die from injuries not related to either occupational or motor-vehicle accidents. At least three studies have found that deaths from injuries were 1.3 to 1.6 times more common among smokers than among nonsmokers. In another study, after controlling for age, sex, race, employment status and alcohol use, people hospitalized with unintentional, non–motor-vehicle, nonburn injuries were 2.0 times more likely than randomly selected controls from the community to be cigarette smokers.

Possible reasons for increased risk of injury. According to Sacks and Nelson[5] there are four possible reasons why smoking increases the risk of injury:

- Direct toxicity: Carbon monoxide or nicotine may have direct toxic effects that increase the risk of injury. Studies have confirmed, for example, that the higher levels of carboxyhemoglobin found in smokers' blood are associated with decreased night vision and lower scores on vision tests.

- Distractibility: The simple act of finding, lighting and holding a cigarette preoccupies a smoker, thereby reducing his or her ability to react to unexpected conditions. In addition, the eye irritation caused by cigarette smoke may distract smokers from their tasks, also increasing their risk of injury.

- Medical conditions associated with smoking that may decrease alertness: Some researchers hypothesize that cancer and heart disease associated with smoking may increase the risk of injury-causing accidents, possibly by decreasing smokers' alertness. Further, because smoking can cause cataracts, it can also decrease vision, thereby increasing the risk of injury.

- Confounding factors, including substance abuse and personality or behavioral characteristics: Smokers are more apt to use alcohol and other drugs, and the use of these substances may increase injury risk. Some studies suggest that smokers are more likely than nonsmokers to be nervous, anxious and emotional—personality characteristics that may predispose them to injury. In addition, smokers are more likely to be risk takers, another factor leading to a greater risk of injury.

References

1 Miller AL. *The U.S. smoking-material fire problem through 1992. The role of lighted tobacco products in fire.* National Fire Protection Association. 1 Batterymarch Park, P.O. Box 9101, Quincy, MA 02269. October 1994.

2 No significant federal legislation has been passed to require "fire-safe cigarettes" that won't ignite bedding, upholstery or clothing if dropped or left unattended.

3 Brison RP. Risk of automobile accidents in cigarette smokers. *Can J Public Health* 1990;81:102–106.

4 Underwood M. *Arch Intern Med* 1992;152:2347–48 (letter).

5 Sacks JJ, Nelson DE. Smoking and injuries: an overview. *Preventive Medicine* 1994;23:515–520.

Tobaccosis: A Twentieth-Century Catastrophe

Just as the fourteenth century will always be remembered as the century when the Black Death killed almost half the population of Europe, so the twentieth century will be long remembered as the century when tobaccosis mortality caused by the smoking, chewing and snuffing of tobacco reached its epidemic zenith in the United States and when tobaccosis killed more than 100 million worldwide.[1]

Unlike the Black Death, quickly recognized by its blackened buboes upon entry to Europe in 1346, tobaccosis has proved an extraordinarily insidious disease entity since the addictive herb causing it was discovered by Columbus and crew in the West Indies in November 1492. Tobacco was disseminated throughout the world during the following centuries and initially was considered a boon to health. It is only now, late in the fifth post–Columbian century of world tobacco experience, that the catastrophic nature and extent of tobacco's depredations have been fully revealed.

Despite the fact that tobacco purveyors have consistently stonewalled all emerging evidence of tobacco's powerful pathogenicity, denying that smoking is the cause of any disease, most adults in developed countries are now aware that smoking causes addiction, lung cancer, emphysema and heart disease. But few are yet aware of the bodywide range and nature of the total spectrum of diseases caused by tobacco, as detailed in the 20 foregoing chapters, because such diseases are treated disparately by clinical specialists and assigned numerous anatomic diagnoses devoid of the unifying term tobaccosis. Hence the basic causative role of tobacco is often missed and disregarded.

In the case of tuberculosis, however, the records of all patients with any manifestation of tubercle bacillus infection are ordinarily labeled tuberculosis. The same is true for histoplasmosis, asbestosis, silicosis, syphilis and AIDS. For analogous use of the holistic term tobaccosis, many physicians and the public must improve their understanding of nicotine addiction, tobacco's many poisons and its pathogenic mechanisms, as detailed here:

- Nicotine occurs naturally in the tobacco plant. Inhaling smoke is the fastest and most efficient way of getting nicotine to the brain (20 seconds), where it acts through specialized receptors. When these receptors signal the presence of nicotine, a wide range of physical reactions occur: Heart rate and blood pressure rise, peripheral circulation slows, skin temperature drops, hormones affecting the central nervous system are released and brain waves change. These many physiological effects produce a "rush" that most smokers find pleasurable—with habitual use leading to dependence and compulsive abuse, physiological and psychological distress upon discontinuance, and a tendency to recidivism among former smokers. Cigarette smoking is now the most serious and widespread form of addiction in the world.[2]

- Burning tobacco generates smoke containing thousands of noxious products, including the addictive drug nicotine, nitriles, aldehydes, hydrogen cyanide, benzopyrenes, phenols, carbon monoxide and the radioisotope polonium 210—an alpha particle emitter many times more mutagenic than equivalent dosage of x-rays. The combination of an addictive substance (nicotine) with polonium 210 and other potent mutagens has made tobacco the foremost human poison of the twentieth century.[1]

- When tobacco smoke is inhaled deeply into the lungs, most of the tars contained in the smoke are captured and retained by the respiratory mucus that coats the lungs. Immediately soluble components are then promptly absorbed into the pulmonary circulation and conveyed by the systemic circulation throughout the body. Less soluble tars trapped by the mucus are raised by ciliary action and coughing to the pharynx, then swallowed and passed to the esophagus, stomach, intestine, portal circulation and liver. The chronic inhalation of tobacco smoke exposes the entire body—every tissue and cell—to powerful mutagens and carcinogens, thus hastening the malignant cellular evolutionary process and resulting in the accelerated occurrence of the broad spectrum of cancers, degenerative diseases, and other diseases constituting tobaccosis.[1,3]

Tobaccosis denotes, collectively, all those diseases resulting from the smoking, chewing and snuffing of tobacco and the breathing of tobacco smoke.[1] *These include nicotine addiction; cancers of the mouth, nasopharynx, larynx, trachea, bronchi, lungs, esophagus, stomach, liver, pancreas, kidney, bladder, prostate, cervix and brain; colorectal cancer; leukemia; atherosclerosis of the cardiovascular system, including coronary heart disease (with ischemia and infarction), cardiomyopathy, aortic and other aneurysms, cerebrovascular hemorrhages and blockages, renal failure and peripheral vascular disease; emphysema; chronic obstructive pulmonary disease; pneumonia; childhood asthma; peptic ulcer disease and regional ileitis; cirrhosis of the liver; immunological deficiencies and failures of endocrine and metabolic functions; cataracts; osteoporosis; optic neuropathy; infertility; fetal and neonatal deaths and child disabilities; and more.* Although tobaccosis is usually not the only cause of these many diseases, it is an important contributing cause, and often the dominant cause.

The great multiplicity of diseases caused by tobacco and the usual lengthy latent interval from initiation of tobacco exposure to serious disease and death have greatly obscured the important causative role of tobacco for many of the diseases listed. Furthermore, many clinical and epidemiological studies have failed to obtain adequate quantitive data concerning lifetime exposure to tobacco; hence, the powerful causative role of tobacco is often obscured. If every practicing physician and clinic would routinely obtain a quantitative history of each patient's *lifetime* tobacco experience, then the role of tobacco causality for the diseases and deaths listed would be much better understood. This can readily be done by charting usual levels of smoking by age.[4]

Tobacco is the juggernaut killer among all addiction killers in the United States. It caused approximately five million deaths in the decade of the 80s, compared with one million deaths from alcohol, 350,000 deaths from other addictive substances and 90,000 deaths from AIDS. During the 90s, annual U.S. mortality from tobaccosis has remained close to a half million deaths, with the decreasing mortality from cardiovascular disease offset by increasing mortality from lung cancer, mainly among women (see Table 2, page 174).[5]

Worldwide, annual deaths from tobaccosis have risen above three million, responsive to large increases in global cigarette consumption during recent decades, especially in less developed countries.[1,6] Altogether we are witnessing one of the great tragedies in human history—a burgeoning global pandemic of tobaccosis mortality caused by greedy promotion of tobacco sales and increasing addictive use of the substance despite widespread knowledge of its deadly effects.

REIMERT THOROLF RAVENHOLT, M.D., M.P.H.
President
Population Health Imperatives
P. O. Box 85120
Seattle, Washington

References

1 Ravenholt RT. Tobacco's global death march. *Population and Development Review.* 1990;16:213–239.

2 Pollin W, Ravenholt RT. Tobacco addiction and tobacco mortality: Implications for death certification. *JAMA.* 1984;252:2849–2854.

3 Ravenholt RT. Malignant cellular evolution: An analysis of the causation and prevention of cancer. *Lancet.* 1966;96:523–526.

4 Ravenholt RT. Charting lifetime smoking experience. *World Health Forum.* 1982;2:860–864.

5 Ravenholt RT. Tobacco's impact on twentieth century U.S. mortality patterns. *American Journal of Preventive Medicine.* 1985;1:4–17.

6 Peto R, Lopez AD, Boreham J, Thun M, Heath, Jr., C. *Mortality from Smoking in Developed Countries 1950–2000: Indirect Estimates from National Vital Statistics.* Oxford: Oxford University Press; 1994:211.

TABLE 2: TOBACCOSIS DEATHS ATTRIBUTED TO CIGARETTES AND OTHER TOBACCO USE, UNITED STATES, 1993

By Anatomic Site or Nature of Disease, International Classification of Diseases (ICD Numbers)

	Number of deaths in category	Deaths attributed to tobacco
A) Cancers:		
Lip, oral cavity, pharynx (140–149)	8,241	4,730
Digestive organs (150–159)	124,466	24,893
Respiratory organs (160–165)	154,183	133,060
Breast (174–175)	43,910	3,952
Genital and urinary (179–189)	82,162	19,719
Other and unspecified sites (170–173, 190–199)	65,315	6,270
Lymphatic and hematopoietic (200–203)	32,097	7,703
Leukemia (204–208)	19,530	4,687
Other neoplasms (210–239)	7,441	1,860
Total cancer deaths, United States, 1993	537,345	
Cancer deaths attributed to tobacco use		206,874
Percentage of cancer deaths due to tobaccosis		*38.5%*
B) Cardiovascular diseases:		
Ischemic heart disease (410–414)	490,063	117,615
Cerebrovascular disease (430–438)	150,108	43,231
Other vascular diseases	307,917	73,900
Total cardiovascular disease deaths	948,088	
Cardiovascular deaths attributed to tobacco use		234,746
Percentage of cardiovascular deaths due to tobaccosis		*24.8%*
C) Other selected diseases:		
Pneumonia and influenza (480–487)	82,820	15,901
Chronic obstructive pulmonary disease (490–496)	101,077	58,119
Chronic liver disease/cirrhosis (571)	25,209	3,781
Infant deaths (760–779)	15,097	3,623
External causes of injury (fires, etc.)	90,523	4,526
Miscellaneous and ill-defined diseases	26,540	3,981
Total deaths, other selected diseases	341,266	
Deaths attributed to tobacco use, other selected diseases		89,931
Total deaths, U.S., 1993	**[2,268,553]***	
Estimated tobaccosis deaths, U.S. 1993		**531,551**
Percentage of total deaths attributed to tobaccosis		*23.4%*

*[Includes categories not listed above]

Data from *Monthly Vital Statistics Report,* February 29, 1996. Tobacco mortality estimates by R. T. Ravenholt, M.D., M.P.H., and E. M. Whelan, D.Sc., M.P.H., derived from *Advance Report of Final Mortality Statistics,* 1993, CDC, Atlanta, GA 30333 and by updating mortality estimates made in references 1, 2 and 5 (see page 173) and in Ravenholt, RT. Cigarette smoking: Magnitude of the hazard. *Am J Public Health* 1964;54:1923–1925.

EPILOGUE

Since this book was first published last fall (1996), the cigarette industry has been beset by crisis after crisis: new revelations mount about the companies' fraud and deceit and legal actions by state governments appear to be driving the industry into making a "grand deal" in which it would finally be forced to pay for the harm done by its product. Or would it?

The April 1997 settlement between the states and the Liggett Group, the smallest of the major cigarette companies, may be the prototype for a plan that all the major tobacco companies would join. The settlement between the Liggett Group and the attorneys general of twenty-two states raised the possibility of congressional or court-sanctioned protection for the tobacco industry. The crux of such a plan is a trade-off in which the industries pay money to the states in return for immunity from all lawsuits—and the opportunity to do business as usual.

According to the terms of the deal, Liggett will publicly admit that cigarettes are addictive; give court access to internal industry documents; and pay 25 percent of their pre-tax income, fully tax-deductible for twenty-five years, to a settlement fund. In return, they have been granted much more than immunity from public lawsuits related to recouping Medicare and Medicaid costs. In a little known link to the settlement, the presiding judge, on questionable legal grounds, exempted Liggett from all litigation, public and private, nationwide, As a result, consumers are now barred from pursuing individual litigation against the company.

As we go to press, the media reports that the two largest companies in the tobacco industry—Philip Morris Companies and RJR Nabisco Holdings Corporation—are seeking a similar deal with Congress that will shield them from the current barrage of litigation, and particularly from the threat of both individual and class-action lawsuits. Under the terms of the proposed deal, the cigarette industry would pay $250 billion into an industry fund to be used, in great part, toward individual smokers' claims against cigarette companies. The industry would also agree to accept FDA regulation and some minor advertising restrictions. In return for these concessions, the industry would receive what, for them, would be a priceless gift: the complete immunity to all current and future litigation.

Although the proposed agreement may appear to punish the cigarette industry, what is currently known about the deal suggests that it will benefit only the cigarette manufacturers and the attorneys who negotiate it. The $250 billion payment over twenty-five years in compensatory damages may appear to be a significant setback for the industry; in reality, however:

1. Compensatory damages, unlike punitive damages, are tax deductible. This reduces the economic impact on the companies by half or more.

2. What the industry would get in return—immunity from lawsuits—would tremendously enhance the value of cigarette stocks.

Such a deal is thus a win-win scenario for the tobacco companies. (Tobacco stock prices soared even on the rumor of a settlement.)

The ever-present threat of litigation is a strong motivation to manufacturers to keep up-to-date and to be forthcoming on the medical risks of their products. If that threat is removed, the tobacco companies have no incentive to act responsibly or to make their products safer.

Also as we go to press, a North Carolina judge has ruled that the Food and Drug Administration does have the authority to regulate nicotine as a drug and cigarettes as a drug delivery system. FDA regulation would be an annoyance to the cigarette industry but would have little effect on the sale of tobacco products. Furthermore, the tobacco industry is well aware that it can easily circumvent any regulatory move the FDA may make against it. If, for example, the, FDA moved to ban cigarette advertising in magazines read primarily by children and teenagers (as has been proposed), the industry could simply redefine "cigarette ad" and place surrogate ads—ads for promotional items such as Camel shoes, Marlboro hats, and Virginia Slims jackets—in the affected magazines. This is precisely what has happened in countries such as France that have legislated partial or complete bans on cigarette advertising.

So an FDA "win" would not be a significant loss for the cigarette industry and it would not be a major benefit to public health advocates.

Whatever new legal wrangling occurs in the coming months and years, the information in this book shows the fallacy of the oft-heard argument that "everyone knows the dangers of smoking"—the claim that the cigarette industry has perpetually used to defend itself against lawsuits. With that mantra now breaking down in the face of reality, it is no small wonder they are seeking legal cover. The question is, will Congress and the courts allow this?

Cigarette manufacturers have long enjoyed a privileged legal status. The time is overdue for treating cigarette companies as we treat any other American corporation, without the protection of congressional intervention. Lawsuits against cigarette companies should be allowed to proceed unfettered by "deals." No other industry would be given such protection, so why should Congress protect the tobacco industry, the manufacturer of the product that is the leading cause of death in America? If future juries should find cigarette companies guilty of fraud, deception, or failure to warn, the decisions could trigger a cascade of events—none of which would require governmental regulation—that could lead to a natural decline in the prevalence of smoking in America.

Laying out the grim facts as to the harm caused by cigarettes is the key to reducing the pandemic of tobacco-related death and illness. Ultimately, the responsibility to inform the American public as to the dangers of smoking should fall neither to independent scientists nor the government, but to those who produce and sell the product. In the meantime, we hope this volume will help to inform both the citizenry and the national leadership as to why it is so important—indeed, America's number one health priority—that the tobacco industry assume this responsibility.

INDEX

0215
1061